Progress in Transfusion Medicine

Progress in Transfusion Medicine

Volume 3

Edited by

John D. Cash

National Medical Director, Scottish National
Blood Transfusion Service, Edinburgh, UK

CHURCHILL LIVINGSTONE
EDINBURGH LONDON MELBOURNE AND NEW YORK 1988

CHURCHILL LIVINGSTONE
Medical Division of Longman Group UK Limited

Distributed in the United States of America by
Churchill Livingstone Inc., 1560 Broadway, New York,
N.Y. 10036, and by associated companies, branches
and representatives throughout the world.

First published 1988

ISBN 0-443-03721-3
ISSN 0268 2613

British Library Cataloguing in Publication Data
Progress in transfusion medicine.
   Vol. 3
   1. Blood — Transfusion
   615'.65   RM171

**The Library of Congress has cataloged this
serial as follows:**
Progress in transfusion medicine. — Vol. 1- — Edinburgh; New
   York: Churchill Livingstone, 1986-
      v.: ill.; 25 cm.
   Annual.
   ISSN 0268-2613 = Progress in transfusion medicine.

   1. Blood—Transfusion—Periodicals.
   [DNLM: 1. Blood Transfusion—periodicals.   W1PR684E]
RM171.P76   615'.65'005—dc19   86-641477
   AACR 2   MARC-S

Library of Congress
                                                    [8705]

Printed in Great Britain at The Bath Press, Avon

Preface

Over the last five years there has been increasing concern, worldwide, that the integration of blood transfusion services into local and national health care services is less than satisfactory. A committee of experts of the Council of Europe came to the same conclusion and noted that in many countries there is little evidence of co-ordination, but much evidence of fragmentation of effort and inadequate clinical monitoring of the use of costly and scarce human blood resources. These could lead to inappropriate treatment of individual patients with attendant waste and possible health risks. The committee recommended that there was an urgent need for the creation of national and community based blood transfusion centres which should be centres of excellence in a newly created specialty, transfusion medicine, and made specific proposals with regard to the training of doctors who would work in such centres.

Colleagues in the United States of America have shared these concerns and the National Institute of Health is currently investing significant resources into developing a Transfusion Medicine Academic Award Programme.

The arrival of a new annual publication entitled *Progress in Transfusion Medicine* is a direct result of this rapidly growing worldwide interest. Whilst the views of individual chapter authors may not necessarily be shared by the editor, the topics covered will mirror the extensive curriculum proposed by the European Committee of Experts. It can be anticipated that particular, but not exclusive, attention will be placed upon the clinical aspects of transfusion practice.

Edinburgh, 1988   J. D. C.

Contributors

Tasnim Azim MB BS
Research Assistant, Department of Virology, Royal Postgraduate Medical School, London, UK

William L. Bayer MD
Director, Community Blood Center of Greater Kansas City, Missouri, USA

William I. Bensinger BSc MD
Assistant Professor of Medicine, University of Washington, and Assistant Member, Fred Hutchinson Cancer Research Center, Seattle, Washington, USA

David Beverley MA MB ChB MRCP
Senior Registrar in Paediatrics, St James's University Hospital, Leeds, UK

Marcela Contreras BSc MD
Director, North London Blood Transfusion Centre, Edgware, Middlesex; Senior Lecturer in Haematology, St Mary's Hospital, London, UK

Dorothy H. Crawford MB BS PhD MRCPath
Senior Lecturer in Virology, Royal Postgraduate Medical School, London, UK

Geoff L. Daniels PhD
Member of Scientific Staff, MRC Blood Group Unit, London, UK

J. S. Finlayson PhD
Associate Director for Science Division of Blood and Blood Products, Food and Drug Administration, Bethesda, Maryland, USA

S. A. Gould PhD
Associate Professor in Surgery, University of Chicago, Pritzker School of Medicine; Attending Surgeon, Michael Reese Hospital, Chicago, Illinois, USA

Patricia E. Hewitt MRCP MRCPath
Deputy Director, North London Blood Transfusion Centre, Middlesex, UK

E. R. Huehns PhD MD MRCS
Professor and Chairman of Department of Haematology, University College Hospital Medical School, London, UK

W. John Judd FIMLS MIBiol
Associate Professor of Medical Technology, Department of Pathology, University of Michigan, Ann Arbor, Michigan, USA

Harvey G. Klein MD
Chief, Department of Transfusion Medicine, National Institutes of Health, Bethesda, Maryland, USA

Hugh M. Moores BSc AFIMA
Principal Computing Officer, Department of Clinical Pharmacology, University of Edinburgh

Gerald S. Moss MD
Professor in Surgery, Pritzker School of Medicine, University of Chicago; Chairman, Department of Surgery, Michael Reese Hospital and Medical Center, Chicago, Illinois, USA

Harold A. Oberman MD
Professor of Pathology, Head, Section of Clinical Pathology, and Director of Blood Bank, University of Michigan, Ann Arbor, Michigan, USA

Anna Parravicini ScD
Chief Technologist, Centro Transfusionale e di Immunologia dei Trapianti, Ospedale Policlinico, Milano, Italy

Paolo Rebulla MD
Section Head, Centro Transfusionale e di Immunologia dei Trapianti, Ospedale Policlinico, Milano; Associate Professor of Hematology, University of Milano, Italy

A. L. Rosen PhD
Physiologist, Department of Surgery, Michael Reese Hospital and Medical Center, Chicago; Research Associate (Assistant Professor), Pritzker School of Medicine, University of Chicago, Illinois, USA

Hansa L. Sehgal BSMT
Research Associate, Department of Surgery, Michael Reese Hospital, Chicago, Illinois, USA

Lakshman R. Sehgal PhD
Director of Surgical Research, Michael Reese Hospital and Medical Center; Assistant Professor, Pritzker School of Medicine, University of Chicago, Illinois, USA

Girolamo Sirchia MD
Director, Centro Transfusionale e di Immunologia dei Trapianti, Ospedale Policlinico, Milano, Italy

Cees Th. Smit Sibinga MD PhD
Medical Director, Red Cross Bloodbank, Gröningen, The Netherlands

G. E. Tegtmeier PhD
Director of Research, Community Blood Center of Greater Kansas City, Missouri, USA

R. deWoskin BS
Department of Surgery, Michael Reese Hospital and Medical Center, Chicago, Illinois, USA

Contents

M. Contreras   P. Hewitt

The cross-match

INTRODUCTION

Landsteiner's discovery of the ABO blood groups was first put to practical application in blood transfusion by Ottenberg (1908). Since that time there has been a constant modification of the apparently simple concept of the mixing of donor's and recipient's blood (the cross-match) which Ottenberg introduced and which has become standard practice in the provision of safe blood transfusion. More recently, years of constant striving to improve the sensitivity of the cross-match procedure have been reversed by the trend to simplify, abbreviate, or even in certain special circumstances dispense with the cross-match, in conjunction with improved antibody screening techniques.

The first cross-match

In the 19th century, transfusion of blood was associated with such frequent adverse reactions that it became fashionable to explore the use of other fluids (such as electrolyte solutions) for transfusion. However, Landsteiner's discovery was recognised as being of importance in explaining the occurrence of adverse reactions to blood transfusion and Ottenberg was encouraged by his superior Weil to implement a practical method of matching donor and recipient blood, which represented the first efforts in pretransfusion testing.

THE MINOR CROSS-MATCH

Ottenberg's method involved the mixing of donor's red cells and recipient's serum with observation for lysis and agglutination. This represented the 'major cross-match'. The reverse technique, the 'minor cross-match', was recognised as being of relatively little significance (Ottenberg & Kaliski 1913) – a salutary thought when it is considered that it was accepted as part of standard practice in most countries including the United States where it was only finally deemed unnecessary in the 1976 edition of the *Standards* of the American Association of Blood Banks. One justification for continuing this procedure was that it would prevent transfusion of group O blood with high titre of isoantibodies to patients of other ABO groups. The main explanation for its downfall, however, was the introduction and gradual acceptance during the 1950s and 1960s of screening tests on donor serum for the presence of unexpected antibodies. By the mid 1960s such screening of donor serum was becoming a standard procedure, and the necessity for the minor cross-match disappeared although a high proportion of blood banks continued the practice until the late 1970s. This persistence was despite convincing evidence by Mohn in 1961 showing the absence of adverse effects attributable to transfer of donor antibodies in a series of 76 380 units of whole blood transfused. Mohn's observations were supported by Giblett in 1977, who pointed out the need to avoid giving group O whole blood to non-O recipients and blood from donors with anti-D to antenatal patients or infants suffering from Rh haemolytic disease of the newborn. She stated that there was no need for elaborate tests to screen donor blood for red cell alloantibodies other than anti-D since the incidence of clinically important antibodies in donors is rare and, if present, they are usually weak and unlikely to cause haemolytic transfusion reactions in recipients carrying the relevant antigens.

THE MAJOR CROSS-MATCH

Between 1907 and the mid 1940s the role of the cross-match in the prevention of haemolytic transfusion reactions was limited. Improvements and refinements in technique included the introduction of blood typing, but tests were still carried out at room temperature and all haemagglutination reactions involved saline ('complete') agglutinating antibodies. The cross-match did not advance further until the 1940s. It was then that 'incomplete' or 'blocking antibodies' were recognised independently by Race (1944) and Wiener (1944); and methods for their detection soon followed. These included the introduction of polymers such as albumin to potentiate haemagglutination, the antiglobulin technique (Coombs et al 1945) and treatment of red cells with proteolytic enzymes. The importance of performing these tests at 37°C was also realised by a few workers at this time. In the 1950s tube tests became standard practice, and the availability of good quality reagent red cells led to the introduction of pretransfusion antibody screening of the donor's serum. Surprisingly, antibody screening of the recipient's serum was not introduced until much later. Further increases in the sensitivity of techniques followed, with the introduction of centrifugation to speed agglutination tests, enhancement of the rate of uptake of antibody by red cells with the use of low ionic strength saline solutions (Löw & Messeter 1974) and more recent refinements such as the manual polybrene test (Steane et al 1985). The constant improvements in the sensitivity of both pretransfusion antibody screening of the donor's serum and of the major cross-match led to the recognition, in the 1950s and 1960s, of a number of previously unknown or undescribed red cell antigens and antibodies. There was increasing pressure to practice techniques which would detect every 'incompatibility' in the test-tube, and although the aim was to provide safer blood transfusion it gradually became evident that some of the testing might be unnecessary, not cost-effective and detrimental to the recipient due to unnecessary delays in the provision of compatible blood. Thus, over recent years the discussion has concentrated on the balance between the need to detect clinically significant antibodies in a recipient's serum – thus avoiding the transfusion of blood which would cause haemolytic reactions – and the logistics, cost and effort which should be spent on this task. Much of the debate has taken place in the last five years, and recommendations and accepted practices are still undergoing constant revision. One aspect however, which is reaching universal acceptance is that the term 'cross-match' is outdated and is an inaccurate description of the test carried out. Since the procedure now involves only half of the original 'cross test' as described in the early part of this century, there is good reason to abandon the term 'cross-match' and replace it with the title 'compatibility test', which is just one part of accepted modern pretransfusion testing.

Optimum temperature for the cross-match

Early workers used incubations at room temperature for their cross-match techniques. Testing at 37°C was not general practice until the mid 1940s and the recognition of the significance of IgG antibodies. An incubation phase at 37°C was then added to the cross-match technique and to the increasingly accepted pretransfusion antibody screening of donor's serum. In the early 1970s the *Standards* of the American Association of Blood Banks required that laboratories should employ techniques in pretransfusion testing which would detect 'all agglutinating, coating and haemolyzing antibodies in donor and recipient serum'. There was no consideration as to whether all such antibodies were of clinical significance.

Inevitably, the next few years following the 1974 directive of the AABB were filled with discussion and concern that many of the antibodies detected in either donor's or recipient's serum were of no clinical significance whatever. Their detection simply led to unnecessary work, expense, worry for the recipient and inconvenience, if not danger, for the individual who suffered postponement of surgery or blood transfusion while 'room temperature only' antibodies were further investigated. Giblett (1977) attacked the use of room temperature techniques in pre-transfusion testing in both antibody screening of blood donors and compatibility testing. Her opinion was supported by a number of reports, including early work by Mollison (1959). For several years Mollison and co-workers showed by in vivo survival studies that antibodies reacting below 30°C caused no accelerated destruction of red cells in vivo and recommended that such antibodies be ignored for practical blood transfusion purposes (see Mollison 1983). Most naturally occurring antibodies that are not reactive at 37°C are IgM, and there is no evidence that they change into IgG antibodies reactive at 37°C following the transfusion of blood containing the appropriate antigen. Furthermore, antibodies which are only doubtfully active at 37°C will not cause any serious degree of destruction of red blood cells which are transfused therapeutically, although such antibodies could increase in potency following transfusion of red cells, leading to a delayed haemolytic transfusion reaction.

It seems strange that in the face of the above evidence, there is still discussion about room temperature tests. In 1978 the AABB deemed room temperature testing unnecessary for the purpose of both antibody screening and compatibility testing. Yet in the United Kingdom a large proportion of laboratories (Holburn, personal communication) still persist in this historical and wasteful technique for reasons which do not hold up to close examination. There is no advantage to be gained by the knowledge of the presence of antibodies inactive at 30°C, and it is time that room temperature testing in the antibody screen is consigned to where it belongs – the history books.

PRETRANSFUSION ANTIBODY SCREENING

Pretransfusion antibody screening is not a new concept, although judging by the debate in the last ten years we might be excused for thinking that this is so. In 1955 Kissmeyer-Nielsen published a review of irregular blood group antibodies found in 17 011 random blood samples from donors, patients, and pregnant women. He found that 1.28% of sera contained one or more antibodies. Blood grouping and antibody screening were performed routinely on all patients for whom blood was cross-matched. Screening continued in his laboratory with variation in the techniques used as new methods were described (albumin, papain, trypsin, bromelin, indirect antiglobulin methods). In 1965 a further report by his group indicated that 2.1% of individuals possessed one or more irregular antibodies. Half of these antibodies were of anti-D specificity, and 15% belonged to the Lewis system. In the study it was also found that a significant proportion of the anti-E and anti-c antibodies were revealed only by a two-stage papain technique, and although most of such antibodies were weak, there were a number of strong antibodies not detected by the indirect antiglobulin method. Kissmeyer-Nielsen commented that only 2.6% of the total antibodies found were detected during cross-matching, but not during antibody screening, which 'confirms the efficiency of the antibody screening procedures'. The conclusion reached by this study was that if grouping was not accompanied by antibody screening tests, then 'a reliable compatibility test is of crucial importance to detect "all" irregular blood group anti-bodies'; a two-stage enzyme technique should be included to supplement the saline room temperature test (to check ABO compatibility) and the indirect antiglobulin test. Kissmeyer-Nielsen recommended antibody screening as a safe procedure which would provide increased security against haemolytic transfusion reactions when used as a supplement to ABO-compatibility tests.

In the early 1960s, workers in the United States, notably Grove-Rasmussen (1964) questioned the need for an antiglobulin test in the cross-match if it had been incorporated in antibody screening with negative results. Furthermore, there was argument that pretransfusion antibody screening of a recipient's serum was adequate to detect virtually all clinically significant red cell alloantibodies, and that compatibility testing was not essential. For many years, the American authorities (AABB and College of American Pathologists) insisted that pretransfusion testing of recipient's serum should include both antibody screening and cross-matching against any unit of blood which might be transfused – and in 1970 the AABB stipu-lated that both procedures should include an antiglobulin test. Inevitably, questions began to be raised as to the necessity for this 'double' testing which increased laboratory costs and workload significantly without producing a great deal of benefit for the patient. Moreover, many patients have blood cross-matched in the expectation, no matter how small, that blood might be transfused – and only a proportion do in fact require a blood transfusion. This fact renders the cross-match inefficient – blood is earmarked for an individual patient who may have a very small chance indeed of actually requiring the reserved blood. If, in a given hospital, a large proportion of the cross-matches are carried out for these less than certain transfusions, there is the inevitable result that blood reaches its expiry date without ever being used – having been set aside for two, three, or more patients during its shelf-life without a real likelihood that it will ever be transfused.

Even though there is the remote possibility that a cross-match may reveal an antibody to a low frequency antigen which has not been detected in anti-body screening, and it acts as a second check on accuracy, the second half of the 1970s saw a great interest awakened in the abbreviation of the cross-match. This contrasted with a report by Pineda (1978) pointing out that, despite the advances in serological techniques, compatibility tests did not detect all antibodies which are capable of causing a haemolytic reaction. His plea was for 'better and more sensitive cross-match techniques' to ensure compatibility in situations where primary immunisation had already occurred, but circulating antibody was not detectable. Hence, the late 1970s saw an apparent conflict between the perceived need to detect all clinically significant antibodies and the need to avoid expensive, time-consuming laboratory practices. Inevitably, the debate leads to an assessment of what is considered cost-effective, and what is a reasonable risk.

ABBREVIATION OF THE CROSS-MATCH

The first stimulus towards abbreviation of the cross-match came from two reports published in 1976 by Mintz et al and Friedman et al. These two groups independently reported a new concept for preoperative ordering of blood which came to be known as the 'maximum surgical blood order schedule' (MSBOS). They proposed that where a patient was to undergo planned surgery which had a low likelihood of requiring blood transfusion then there was no necessity to cross-match blood for the patient, providing that ABO, Rh(D) typing and antibody screening had been performed (and that the screening revealed no clinically significant antibodies). Confirmation of the basic safety of this approach was given by Boral & Henry (1977). They examined their own experience with 12 848 blood samples using the 'type and screen' as well as the cross-match during 1975. With a two-cell antibody screening test they detected 96.11% of the 283 antibodies present in 247 patients. The antibody screen failed to detect antibodies directed against low frequency antigens which were subsequently revealed in cross-matching. Using this information, they were able to calculate that if only typing and screening had been performed, its efficacy in the prevention of the transfusion of serologically incompatible units would have been 99.99%. Their conclusion was that the type and screen was a safe alternative to a two unit cross-match when considering a surgical procedure not usually requiring transfusion. They did not propose that the cross-match should be abandoned, and in fact recommended that a cross-match *should* be performed for all procedures which are fully expected to require blood. The type and screen procedure rapidly became popular, and the benefit it confers by conserving limited resources for those patients who will usually require blood is not challenged.

It is perhaps not surprising that the natural sequel of the above was the argument that if the type and screen procedure was safe for selected patients, it should be safe for all potential recipients. The impetus came from the United States, where cost containment is perhaps a more immediate consideration than for many other countries (see Chapter 9). Several different workers in the United States set about justifying this approach by showing how safe antibody screening is, when used as a pretransfusion test for the presence of clinically significant antibodies. The late 1970s saw a number of reports which summarised large studies focussing on the safety of a type and screen procedure for all patients, and the abbreviation, or even elimination of the cross-match.

The common concept at this time was that if a pretransfusion antibody screen was negative, the antiglobulin phase of the cross-match could be omitted. Indeed, it appeared to some that the cross-match added little to patient safety from the point of view of recognition of clinically significant antibodies, although it was still necessary to retain a procedure which would detect inadvertent ABO incompatibility. In 1980 the regulations of the

AABB and the FDA required that an antiglobulin technique was used in both antibody screening and cross-matching. Following reports such as those by Mintz et al (1982) and Oberman et al (1982) it was apparent that the omission of the antiglobulin technique from the cross-match would not seriously jeopardise the safety of blood transfusion, although the risk was higher than that stated by Boral and Henry. A number of antibodies of doubtful or no clinical significance were detected in a cross-match in patients whose serum showed a negative antibody screen, but the number of clinically significant antibodies so revealed was small. In view of the rarity of such antibodies it was felt that the risk to the patient was very slight indeed, while the benefits in the form of saving on time and money were immense. Heistø (1979) performed concurrent antibody screenings (two cells by antiglobulin technique and one R_1R_2 cell by the enzyme technique) and compatibility tests on 23 857 patients to supply 73 407 units of blood. The only antibodies detected by the antiglobulin phase of the cross-match which were missed by the antibody screening tests were one weak anti-Le^a and two very weak antibodies which defied identification. Oberman and his co-workers calculated in 1981 that the cost of antiglobulin testing in the cross-match in their laboratory was $80 000, and the result of such testing was to reveal four otherwise unsuspected clinically significant antibodies in 32 339 patients. Two of these antibodies were directed against low frequency antigens, so that the chance of the patients in question receiving incompatible blood would have been extremely small. It was only a matter of time before the FDA and AABB allowed the omission of the antiglobulin phase of the cross-match, providing that it had been incorporated in a pretransfusion antibody screen which was negative. Garratty in 1986 calculated that 'one antibody of potential clinical significance might not be detected in every 17 000 compatibility tests if the antiglobulin phase of the cross-match is not performed'. He compared this risk with some of the other quantifiable risks to which patients might be exposed during a hospital stay and felt that a 1 in 17 000 risk of not detecting an antibody (which could cause shortened survival of transfused red cells but would be unlikely to cause mortality in the recipient) was acceptable compared with other potential risks.

THE ROLE OF THE CROSS-MATCH

It has been generally agreed that the cross-match serves as the final check of serological compatibility between donor and recipient. If it is felt that pretransfusion antibody screening (including an enzyme and antiglobulin technique) will detect the overwhelming majority of clinically significant antibodies, and therefore alert blood bank staff to those recipients who need further testing before the issue of suitable blood, is there any need to cross-match at all for the remainder of recipients? The usual answer is 'yes', because inadvertent selection of a unit of blood which is ABO incompatible with the recipient can be avoided by the addition to the antibody screen of a limited or abbreviated cross-match. The argument now rages – what technique or techniques should be employed in order to guard against this most serious and potentially fatal occurrence? It is worth noting that Rouault (1980) reported that in a 13 month period involving 56 235 cross-matches, two units of blood which were ABO incompatible with their recipients were issued. In each case, however, the cross-match would not have prevented the mistake as the blood was given in error to a patient other than the one for whom it had been cross-matched. Clerical and identification errors still account for a significant proportion of ABO incompatible blood transfusions. Perhaps we should concentrate more on identifying donors and recipients rather than in performing sophisticated tests which will be of no great help to the patient.

It is difficult to estimate the risk due to inadvertent ABO incompatibility if the cross-match were to be eliminated completely. Anecdotal reports such as those of Oberman (1981) point to the need to retain some form of cross-match procedure to guard against clerical or technical errors in ABO typing – which could lead to fatal results. In the early 1980s it was felt to be perfectly acceptable to rely on an 'immediate spin' procedure to confirm ABO compatibility, with a very low risk to the patient of a clinically significant antibody being missed by the antibody screening test. However, Berry-Dortch et al (1985) reported on the unreliability of an immediate spin cross-match to detect significant incompatibility between A_2B donor red cells and group B serum. It has also been documented that incompatibility between group A_2 red cells and group O serum can be missed on an immediate-spin technique. Thus in 1986, argument is again raging about the importance or necessity of an antiglobulin cross-match, which would detect most such ABO incompatibilities – or, alternatively, the need to retest the ABO group of all donor red cells immediately prior to release of blood on the result of an immediate-spin test. The wheel has come full circle and more since the early 1960s.

Mintz et al (1982), in a report of their own experience with clinically significant red cell antibodies detected in a cross-match after a negative antibody screening test calculated that each such antibody cost $5632 (in direct costs) to detect. They compared the small risk resulting from these unexpected antibodies of possible clinical significance to the two far more significant problems in blood transfusion today – incorrect identification of patients' specimens or units of blood, and the 7% incidence (in the United States) of post transfusion hepatitis. They raised the question whether resources were being correctly allocated – but also whether any savings in money or staff time occurring from abbreviation of the cross-match would lead to tangible benefits in other areas.

In the face of all the above arguments it may be a surprise to hear that at least one suggestion has recently been made (Garratty 1986) that the costs of pretransfusion testing might be reduced, and more benefit arise, if antibody screening were to be abandoned, and workers concentrate on the cross-match! It is clear that in this very controversial field, opinion remains very much divided and interest has once more returned to the possibility of adopting new, more sensitive cross-match techniques which will allow detection of clinically significant red cell antibodies without the use of an antiglobulin phase. Steane et al (1985) presented data supporting the use of a manual polybrene technique as a rapid sensitive cross-match test, which when used in conjunction with antibody screening incorporating an indirect antiglobulin technique provided for safe red cell transfusion without the need for a further antiglobulin technique in the cross-match. The benefit of this method was that it proved sensitive in the detection of clinically significant antibodies, but it shared with the immediate spin and LISS techniques the failure to detect all incompatibilities in the ABO system – for example some A_2B red cells tested against group B sera. The conclusion was that there is no substitute for properly performed ABO grouping on both donors and recipients. In their hands, the omission of the antiglobulin phase of the cross-match was associated with minimal risk, and the manual polybrene technique conferred an extra safety over the standard room temperature tests. All patients with negative antibody screens who were likely to be transfused had blood cross-matched using the manual polybrene test, similarly patients not deemed likely to require blood who subsequently needed a transfusion had a manual polybrene cross-match test when the blood was issued. Only if a clinically significant antibody was detected during antibody screening was an antiglobulin technique employed in the cross-match.

From all the above, it can be seen that in 1987 there is no universally accepted combination which will constitute a correct pretransfusion test. While all would agree that it is necessary to perform ABO and Rh(D) typing on both donor and recipient and to select ABO and Rh(D) compatible units of blood for transfusion, there is a variety of opinions as to what else is necessary to ensure a safe blood transfusion. How much can we afford in order to ensure the detection of every potentially significant antibody? Should there be more emphasis on antibody screening – using at least an enzyme and an antiglobulin technique – with efforts made to improve the quality of reagent red cells, and less attention paid to the cross-match? Alternatively, should the direction be towards improved cross-match techniques, bearing in mind that the cross-match is arguably most important as verification of ABO compatibility – since it is discrepancies in this area which are most likely to kill recipients? Should the choice of suitable pretransfusion tests be influenced by the indication for the transfusion – does an 'elective' blood transfusion merit more sophisticated or sensitive techniques than an emergency one? It is already evident that choice will vary from blood bank to blood bank depending upon local conditions – volume of work, experience of staff, proportion of work generated by elective surgical procedures, presence of a blood ordering policy, and not least, cost-effectiveness.

FUTURE DEVELOPMENTS IN THE CROSS-MATCH

The ultimate test of compatibility of transfused red cells is the demonstration of a normal life-span of those cells in the recipient's circulation. Despite all the advances which have been made in in vitro cross-match techniques, there are occasions when it is necessary to perform an in vivo test using isotope labelled red cells – for example where an antibody cannot be demonstrated in the recipient's serum, yet transfused red cells have a diminished survival with characteristics which point towards immune-mediated red cell destruction. Further examples include an antibody reacting with the vast majority of cells of a specificity that is known to only rarely cause premature destruction of transfused red cells, or an antibody reacting with all or most examples of red cells whose specificity cannot be established before transfusion must take place. The drawback of the radio-isotope technique is that the survival of a whole unit of transfused red cells cannot necessarily be accurately predicted from the life-span of 1 ml of the same cells used in the diagnostic test (Mollison 1983). Nevertheless, this technique can be an extremely useful adjunct in the assessment of the exceptionally difficult serological problems, especially those cases in which the antibody causes significant red cell destruction.

Attempts continue to be made to improve the predictive value of both in vivo and in vitro serological testing. One such technique, described by Kickler et al (1985) used an enzyme-linked antiglobulin test (ELAT) method to estimate survival of transfused red cells. This proved to be comparable with the radioisotope technique, and other workers have attempted to produce an automated enzyme-linked immunoassay (ELISA) which will provide a sensitive and objective means of detecting clinically significant red cell antibodies.

Other techniques which have elicited much interest as a means of predicting in vivo red cell destruction are the mononuclear phagocyte assay and assays based on antibody dependent cell-mediated cytotoxicity (ADCC). These techniques depend upon the reaction between sensitized red cells and the monocyte/macrophage system and are supposed to mirror the in vivo mechanisms for destruction and removal of IgG and/or C3 coated red cells. Most methods are based on the binding of IgG antibody-coated red cells to Fc receptors on mononuclear phagocytic cells. Some assays are morphological and measure binding and/or phagocytosis while others (ADCC assays) are radiochemical and measure the extracellular lysis of ^{51}Cr-labelled IgG-coated cells. Initial encouraging results were obtained by Engelfriet when studying patients with autoimmune haemolytic anaemia – adherence and ingestion of sensitized red cells by the monocytes/macrophages in vitro correlated with in vivo red cell destruction.

Unfortunately, there is very little convincing data linking results of this in vitro assay with in vivo studies of red cell survival when dealing with alloantibodies. The test may have a predictive value for an individual patient (Schanfield et al 1981), especially if the patient's own monocytes/macrophages are used in the assay, but there is as yet little support for it to be considered a routine investigation. More recently, Urbaniak et al (1984) and Ouwehand (1984) have shown that there is a significant correlation between the capacity of Rh(D) antibodies to cause haemolytic disease of the newborn and their capacity to mediate a positive ADCC assay.

Thus, 80 years on from the initial concept of the cross-match we have no reliable method which will accurately predict the exact fate of a unit of blood which is to be transfused. There are a variety of options which can be followed in deciding how a laboratory can ensure that blood transfusion is as safe as possible. It is comforting that very few incompatibilities outside the ABO system will lead directly to immediate intravascular haemolysis and will per se cause death of a recipient. But the morbidity of a haemolytic transfusion reaction may become significant when superimposed upon a myriad of other clinical problems in an already severely ill patient. While striving to ensure as far as possible the safety of blood which is issued for transfusion purposes, no worker in the blood transfusion field should forget the mortality and morbidity associated with blood transfusion but arising from errors outside the serology laboratory. While educating ourselves and our staff we must also be constantly informing and educating our colleagues who are making the clinical decisions with regard to blood transfusion, and ensuring that all of us strive to make blood transfusion as safe for the recipient as it can possibly be.

SOME PRACTICAL CONSIDERATIONS

From the preceding discussion it is clear that the transfusion of blood of the same ABO and Rh(D) group as the recipient without pre-transfusion antibody screening or cross-matching is 97–99% safe since, in general, not more than 1–3% of prospective recipients of blood have clinically significant red cell alloantibodies other than the expected ABO antibodies or immune anti-D. We must therefore not lose sight that antibody screening and cross-matching benefit only a small minority of recipients. In pre-transfusion testing that minority at risk will benefit if our techniques are able to detect the majority of clinically significant antibodies, i.e. antibodies capable of causing accelerated intravascular or extravascular destruction of incompatible red cells. Obviously, the percentage of immunized prospective recipients will largely depend on the number of patients with a history of previous transfusions or pregnancies.

In the vast majority of cases in vitro pre-transfusion compatibility tests will predict, with a high degree of confidence, the in vivo outcome of a unit of red cells transfused. However, there are rare exceptions where the sensitivity of serological techniques is not as exquisite as required and there are anecdotal reports of the repeated in vivo destruction of red cells found to be compatible by all techniques in vitro (see Mollison 1983, Davey et al 1980, Baldwin et al 1983). In some of these cases the specificity of an antibody likely to be the culprit of the haemolytic transfusion reaction can be suspected from the patient's phenotype; anti-c was suspected by Davey et al in an R_1R_1 patient with no detectable alloantibodies who showed 1% survival of ^{51}Cr labelled c-positive cells at 24 hours and 80% survival of R_1R_1 cells at 24 hours. Baldwin et al have had a similar experience in an R_2R_2 patient in whom anti-e was not detectable by serological techniques but could only be demonstrated by ^{51}Cr survival studies with e-positive and e-negative cells. We have seen three multitransfused patients (two children with thalassaemia and one woman with myelofibrosis) showing haemolysis of ABO and Rh(D) compatible cells in the absence of serologically detectable antibodies; from the red cell phenotypes we suspected anti-c in two patients and anti-E in one. Normal survival of ^{51}Cr labelled c-negative and E-negative cells respectively led to the subsequent successful transfusion maintenance therapy with cells negative for the 'suspected' antigens. On the other hand, there are those not infrequent cases when the transfusion of red cells apparently incompatible in vitro results in normal survival in vivo. Antibodies such as anti-Ch[a], -Rg[a], -Yk[a], Kn[a], -Xg[a], -Sd[a], -Jr[a], etc do not cause accelerated red cell destruction even though they react at 37°C and are detectable by the indirect antiglobulin test (Tilley et al 1977, Silvergleid et al 1977, Mollison 1983, Baldwin et al 1985).

Clinical significance of red cell alloantibodies in the context of the cross-match

Several factors help to predict whether a given antibody found in pre-transfusion testing will cause accelerated red cell destruction. Most important are the thermal range and specificity of the antibody. As discussed previously, antibodies which fail to react in vitro above 30°C can be ignored for blood transfusion purposes; but the opposite does not hold true since not all antibodies active at 37°C will cause accelerated red cell destruction (see above). Knowledge of the specificity of the antibody will also help in the majority of cases to predict the fate of an incompatible unit of blood transfused; antibodies with ABO, Rh, SsU, K, Fy and Jk specificities cause the vast majority of haemolytic transfusion reactions and cannot be ignored in the selection of compatible blood. There are also some antibody specificities which, from past experience, may or may not cause accelerated red cell destruction, e.g. anti-Yt[a] (see Mollison 1983).

Other factors which help to predict the clinical significance of a red cell alloantibody are: the immunoglobulin class and subclass (IgG3, > IgG1 > IgG2 and 4), the ability of the antibody to fix complement, the nature and number of antigen sites on the red cell surface, the strength and equilibrium constant of the antibody, the volume of blood transfused and the presence of the relevant blood group substance in donor plasma (e.g. Le^a, Le^b substances in donor plasma will neutralize Lewis antibodies) and the activity of the recipient's reticuloendothelial system – splenectomized patients with non-complement binding IgG antibodies may, in some cases, not experience significant destruction of antigen-positive cells (Redman et al 1984).

In the vast majority of cases, previous experience and the knowledge of the factors influencing the clinical significance of an antibody will help to correlate the in vitro characteristics of an antibody with its in vivo behaviour. However, it is well known that an ABO incompatible transfusion is not always fatal. Although it can lead in a small number of cases to death of the recipient within a short time, in most cases it will lead to a severe haemolytic reaction or, in some instances, to decreased red cell survival with no symptoms in the recipient. The same holds true for anti-D and other alloantibodies; reactions range from severe haemolysis to unnoticeable decreased red cell survival.

Guidelines for routine pre-transfusion testing

Although there is no consensus on the ideal pre-transfusion testing, the following guidelines may be considered:

1. ABO and Rh(D) typing of donor and recipient is essential. It is advisable to use two different anti-D reagents but tests for D^u are not recommended.

2. A simple antibody screening on the donor's serum by the collecting facility. This test should be capable of detecting anti-D and potent examples of other clinically significant antibodies. Failure to detect weak red cell alloantibodies is unlikely to cause harm to recipients.

3. An antibody screening test on the recipient's serum using 2–3 individual (unpooled) screening cells, by a sensitive antiglobulin technique at 37°C and an enzyme technique at 37°C (de Silva & Contreras 1985). This will detect the vast majority of antibodies capable of causing haemolytic transfusion reactions. Such antibodies should be identified.

4. For those unimmunized patients with a high probability of being transfused, a simple one-tube major cross-match of units of the same ABO and Rh(D) groups should be performed using an immediate spin technique. The tube should then be incubated at 37°C, read for haemolysis and agglutination and finally carried to the antiglobulin phase using a broad spectrum antiglobulin reagent (containing anti-IgG and anti-complement). The major function of this test is a final check on ABO compatibility but it will also detect incompatibility between donor and recipient due to antibodies to low frequency antigens not present in screening cells (e.g. anti-C^w, anti-Kp^a, anti-Wr^a etc).

5. If the patient's serum contains one or more clinically significant anti-

bodies, antigen negative blood should be cross-matched using the same procedure as in 4. plus the technique by which the antibody/ies react best. This procedure should be carried out in all immunized patients even if the likelihood of being transfused is remote. Moreover, it is not unusual for patients who make one antibody to make several more after repeated transfusions (see Mollison 1983).

6. If the patient has not been immunized and is unlikely to require blood transfusion, the serum should be saved and if blood is needed at short notice, units of the same ABO and Rh(D) groups can be cross-matched by an immediate spin technique.

Special considerations

Unlabelled tubes or incomplete/illegible request forms should not be processed and should not be used for cross-matching. The majority of serious incompatible blood transfusions are the result of identification mistakes or clerical errors.

Uncross-matched blood needs to be transfused only in those rare emergencies when there is no time for a short cross-match. If time allows, a rapid ABO and Rh(D) typing should be performed and blood of the same ABO and Rh(D) group should be given. If the blood group of the recipient is unknown, group O, Rh(D) negative red cells should be issued or, failing this, group O Rh-negative whole blood with low titre anti-A,B. Once the patient has been grouped, it is advisable to switch to group-specific blood provided that only 2–3 units of group O blood have been given and that a fresh post-transfusion specimen from the patient shows compatibility.

Massive transfusion. If one whole blood volume has been transfused in a short period of time, it is wasteful to continue cross-matching blood; subsequent units can be given on the basis of an ABO and Rh(D) check or of an immediate spin cross-match.

Previously immunized patients who now show a negative antibody screen should have antigen-negative blood cross-matched if the antibody/ies found in the past was in the category known to cause accelerated red cell destruction. It is not unusual for Kidd antibodies to disappear from the recipient's serum shortly after the antigenic stimulus and to quickly reappear and cause delayed haemolytic transfusion reactions after a challenge with antigen-positive blood.

Repeated transfusions may lead to secondary responses in patients previously immunized by transfusion or pregnancy. For this reason, the serum sample used for cross-matching should be as fresh as possible and not older than 48 hours.

Chronic transfusion regimes. Patients requiring long term blood transfusions (e.g. thalassaemics) should have a blood sample taken not more than 48 hours before the next blood transfusion since they may have developed previously unrecognised red cell alloantibodies after the last transfusion episode.

An autocontrol or direct antiglobulin test on the recipient will only be required if the patient has been transfused within the last three weeks, if the antibody screen is positive or if there is a clinical diagnosis of autoimmune haemolytic anaemia (Judd 1986).

Patients with warm autoimmune haemolytic anaemia ideally should not be transfused. If transfusion is unavoidable and the patient has previously been transfused or pregnant, autoabsorbed serum should be used for the cross-match. If the patient has been transfused within the last three months an antibody screen should be performed on the serum as well as on an eluate from the patient's red cells.

Newborn infants should be given ABO and Rh(D) group-specific blood cross-matched with the infant's or the mother's serum. For repeated transfusions, the same serum sample can be used throughout since infants do not make red cell alloantibodies in the neonatal period.

Intrauterine transfusions should be performed with group O Rh-negative cells cross-matched with the mother's serum.

All units and all panel cells incompatible with the patient's serum in vitro. In such cases every effort should be made to try and identify the antibody/ies by a reference laboratory. If an antibody against a high frequency antigen is identified, antigen-negative blood from the National or International panels of Rare Donors should be requested for cross-matching. If the antibody cannot be identified or if there is no time for identification, blood from sibs or close relatives should be cross-matched in the hope of finding compatible units. If all else fails, an in vivo cross-match with 1 ml of ^{51}Cr-labelled cells mixed from two units of ABO and Rh(D) compatible blood should be performed. If the need for blood transfusion is urgent and there is no time to perform a survival study or if the ^{51}Cr test shows decreased red cell survival, cross-match incompatible blood should be given as a life-saving measure.

In vivo cross-match. A one hour post-transfusion survival of 99% ± 5% denotes compatible red cells. We should remember that the survival of 1 ml of ^{51}Cr-labelled cells may in most cases of immune-mediated red cell destruction be much shorter than that of a whole unit of blood (Mollison 1983) and that survival studies, as tests for in vivo compatibility, are of limited value.

In the vast majority of cases, well performed pre-transfusion tests will be able to predict the outcome of a transfusion of red cells. In general, the tests will be negative and will serve no purpose other than reassuring blood bankers and clinicians that the blood they are transfusing is serologically safe. However, the same goal would have been achieved if blood of the same ABO and Rh group as the recipient was transfused without pre- transfusion testing. It is only 1–3% of patients who will benefit from tests that entail specialized and costly serological investigations in the blood bank.

REFERENCES

American Association of Blood Banks 1970 Standards for blood banks and transfusion services, 5th edn. AABB, Arlington

American Association of Blood Banks 1974 Standards for blood banks and transfusion services, 7th edn. AABB, Arlington

American Association of Blood Banks 1978 Standards for blood banks and transfusion services, 9th edn. AABB, Arlington

Baldwin M L, Barrasso C, Ness P M, Garratty G 1983 A clinically significant erythrocyte antibody detectable only by ^{51}Cr survival studies. Transfusion 23: 40–44

Baldwin M L, Ness P M, Barasso C et al 1985 In vivo studies of the long-term ^{51}Cr red cell survival of serologically incompatible red cell units. Transfusion 25: 34–38

Berry-Dortch S, Woodside C h, Boral L I 1985 Limitations of the immediate spin cross-match when used for detecting ABO incompatibility. Transfusion 25: 176–178

Boral L I, Henry J B 1977 The type and screen: a safe alternative and supplement in selected surgical procedures. Transfusion 17: 163–168

Coombs R R A, Mourant A E, Race R R 1945 A new test for the detection of weak and 'incomplete' Rh agglutinins. British Journal of Experimental Pathology 26: 255–266

Davey R J, Gustafson M, Holland P V 1980 Accelerated immune red cell destruction, in the absence of serologically detectable alloantibodies. Transfusion 20: 348–353

de Silva M, Contreras M 1985 Pooled cells vs. individual screening cells in pre-transfusion testing. Clinical and Laboratory Haematology 7: 369–373

Friedman B A, Oberman H A, Chadwick A R, Kingdon K I 1976 The maximum surgical blood use in the United States. Transfusion 16: 380–388

Garratty G 1986 Abbreviating pretransfusion testing. Transfusion 26: 217–219

Giblett E R 1977 Blood group alloantibodies: an assessment of some laboratory practices. Transfusion 17: 299–307

Grove-Rasmussen M, 1964 Routine compatibility testing. Transfusion 4: 200–205

Heistø H 1979 Pretransfusion blood group serology: limited value of the antiglobulin phase of the cross-match when a careful screening test for unsuspected antibodies is performed. Transfusion 19: 761–763

Judd W J, Barnes B A, Steiner E A, Oberman H A, Averill D B, Butch S H 1986 The evaluation of a positive direct antiglobulin test (autocontrol) in pretransfusion testing revisited. Transfusion 26: 220–224

Kickler T S, Smith B, Bell W, Drew H, Baldwin M, Ness P M 1985 Estimation of transfused red cell survival using an enzyme-linked antiglobulin test. Transfusion 25: 401–405

Kissmeyer-Nielsen F, Bastrup-Madsen K, Stenderup A 1955 Irregular blood group antibodies. Danish Medical Bulletin 2: 202–208

Kissmeyer-Nielsen E 1965 Irregular blood group antibodies in 200 000 individuals. Scandinavian Journal of Haematology 2: 331–342

Löw B, Messeter L 1974 Antiglobulin test in low-ionic strength salt solution for rapid antibody screening and cross-matching. Vox Sanguinis 26: 53–61

Mintz P D, Nordine R B, Henry J B, Webb W R 1976 Expected hemotherapy in elective surgery. New York State Journal of Medicine 76: 532–537

Mintz P D, Haines A C, Sullivan M F 1982 Incompatible cross-match following nonreactive antibody detection test: frequency and cause. Transfusion 22: 107–110

Mohn J F, Lambert R M, Bowman H S, Brason F W 1961 Experimental transfusion of donor plasma containing blood-group antibodies into incompatible normal human recipients. I. Absence of destruction of red-cell mass with anti-Rh, anti-Kell and anti-M. British Journal of Haematology 7:112

Mollison P L 1959 Factors determining the relative clinical importance of different blood group antibodies. British Medical Bulletin 15: 92–98

Mollison P L 1983 Blood Transfusion in Clinical Medicine, 7th edn. Blackwell Scientific Publications, Oxford

Oberman H A 1981 The crossmatch. A brief historical perspective. Transfusion: 21: 645–651

Oberman H A, Barnes B A, Steiner E A 1982 Role of the cross-match in testing for serologic incompatibility. Transfusion 22: 12–16

Ottenberg R 1908 Transfusion and arterial anastomosis. Annals of Surgery 47:486

Ottenberg R, Kaliski D J 1913 Accidents in transfusion. Journal of the American Medical Association 61:2138

Ouwehand W H 1984 The activity of IgG1 and IgG3 antibodies in immune mediated destruction of red cells; clinical significance in rhesus haemolytic disease of the newborn. Thesis, Rodopi, Amsterdam

Pineda A A, Taswell H F, Brzica S M 1978 Delayed haemolytic transfusion reaction – an immunologic hazard of blood transfusion. Transfusion 18: 1–7

Race R R 1944 An 'incomplete' antibody in human serum. Nature, London 153: 771–772

Redman M, Devenish A, Gibson M, Win A A, Ward S, Wiener E, Garner S, Contreras M 1984 Anti-U not causing red cell destruction. British Journal of Haematology 58: 1:193

Rouault C L 1980 Appropriate pretransfusion testing. In: Pretransfusion testing for the '80s. American Association of Blood Banks, Washington, p 125–132

Schanfield M S, Stevens J O, Bauman D, 1981 The detection of clinically significant erythrocyte alloantibodies using a mononuclear phagocyte assay. Transfusion 21: 571–576

Silvergleid A J, Wells R F, Hafleigh E B, Korn G, Kellner J J, Grumet F C 1977 Compatibility test using ^{51}chromium-labeled red blood cells in cross-match positive patients. Transfusion 18: 8–14

Steane E A, Steane S M, Montgomery S R, Pearson J R 1985 A proposal for compatibility testing incorporating the manual hexadimethrine bromide (Polybrene) test. Transfusion 25: 540–544.

Tilley C A, Crookston M C, Haddad S A, Shumak K H 1977 Red blood cell survival studies in patients with anti-Ch[a], anti-Yk[a], anti-Ge and anti-Vel. Transfusion 17: 169–172

Urbaniak S J, Greiss M A, Crawford R J, Fergusson M J C 1984 Prediction of the outcome of rhesus haemolytic disease of the newborn: additional information using an ADCC assay. Vox Sanguinis 46: 323–329

Wiener A S 1944 A new test (blocking test) for Rh sensitization. Proceedings of the Society of Experimental Biology 56: 173–176

Untoward reactions to human albumin preparations

SOME GENERAL CONSIDERATIONS

Purified human albumin for intravenous administration is perceived to be a very 'safe' product. If this perception is warranted, the incidence of untoward reactions must be very low, and one may legitimately ask if there exists sufficient information to fill a chapter.

The incidence of *reported* adverse reactions is indeed small – so small, in fact, that a single case continues to justify publication (e.g. Paul et al 1981, Edelman et al 1985, Maher et al 1986). A comprehensive survey published a decade ago (Barker 1976) revealed that approximately 1.5% of the lots of albumin products made by US manufacturers were associated with untoward reactions. In more than half of these cases, only one patient was reported to have reacted adversely to the lot. The present author's recent experience suggests that a similar calculation (viz. total reactions reported divided by total lots produced in a given year) would still yield a value approximating 1.5%, albeit with considerable fluctuation, for the mid-1980s. In view of the difference in sizes of manufacturing lots, however, these numbers may have little meaning. A prospective study in Germany gave an incidence of 0.01% for anaphylactoid reactions to human albumin when the computation was based on the number of reactions *per vial* infused (Ring & Messmer 1977). Perhaps the truest incidence of untoward reactions would be one calculated on the basis of reactions *per treatment*. Under a passive reporting system such as that in the US, the apparent incidence for *all* reactions would probably continue to be below 0.01%, even if this more stringent basis were employed. Owing to both under-reporting of reactions and the uncertainty of the denominator, one would expect the value to embody appreciable error. Nonetheless, these rough estimates give some quantitative justification for the assumption of safety.

In the following sections some of the untoward reactions are described, some underlying causes are listed, and a few potential sources of adversity are enumerated.

SOME GENERAL DEFINITIONS

This chapter is devoted to albumin-containing solutions administered intra-venously for plasma volume expansion. There are, of course, other prep-arations made from human albumin, such as aggregated albumin particles for lung scanning. Furthermore, albumin can be employed for other purposes (e.g. as a carrier or stabilizer in biological products). These, however, are discussed only briefly. The present section is intended to provide some guidelines – general enough to cross national boundaries but not so general as to be useless – that define the major focus of attention. Particular emphasis is placed on characteristics that may be important in understanding the reasons for (or, in some cases, the reasons for lack of) untoward reactions.

Table 2.1   Characteristics of albumin preparations

1. Sterile solutions (membrane-filtered)
2. Usually isotonic
3. Contain sodium chloride
4. No preservative
5. Stabilizer(s), e.g. caprylate
6. Heated 10 h at 60°C
7. Usually fractionated with cold alcohol
8. Available at two concentrations
   a. up to 25%
   b. 5% or less
9. Sometimes (≤5% solution) available at two levels of purity

Albumin preparations for volume expansion are manufactured as isotonic or slightly hypotonic solutions containing sodium chloride. They are ster-ilized by membrane filtration before filling into the final containers. That is, there is no 'terminal sterilization' or bactericidal step once the product has entered this container. Sterility must be maintained by aseptic filling and the integrity of the container-closure system. The products contain no preservative. They do, however, contain one or more stabilizers such as caprylate because they undergo virucidal heating for 10 hours at 60°C. Depending on the manufacturing history, they may also contain endogenous, protein-bound long-chain fatty acids (Yu & Finlayson 1984a). The protein is usually isolated from plasma by a cold-alcohol fractionation process.

In most countries, albumin solutions are available at two concentrations, one high (e.g. 20% or 25%) and one low (5% or less). Moreover, the prod-ucts with the lower concentration may be available at different levels of purity. That is, whereas albumin always constitutes 95%, 96%, or more of the total protein in the high-concentration solutions, those of lower concen-tration may have this degree of purity or appreciably less. For example, in the US, albumin (human) is manufactured as a 25% and a 5% protein solution, and in both the albumin must amount to at least 96% of the total protein. By contrast, in plasma protein fraction (human), which is also a 5% protein solution, albumin may constitute as little as 83% of the total protein. Analogous products, e.g. stable plasma protein solution (SPPS) and Pasteurisierte Plasmaprotein-Lösung (PPL), are available in other countries. Compounding the complexity, however, is the fact that, depending on the specifications of the national pharmacopeia or manufacturing decisions, products labelled as 'plasma protein fraction' (PPF), PPL, etc. may actually be solutions of highly purified (i.e. ≥ 95% pure) albumin.

In this chapter, 'albumin' is used to designate the more purified preparations, regardless of concentration. When the discussion deals with the products of lower purity, specific nomenclature is used and the differences are indicated. 'Albumin preparations' is a general expression that includes both categories.

TYPES OF REACTIONS: SYMPTOMS

Although, as indicated above, untoward reactions to albumin preparations are infrequent, certain types of responses are found in most compilations of symptoms (Ring et al 1974, Barker 1976, Ring & Messmer 1977, Quast et al 1981). These are listed below, along with some other observations, generally in order of their frequency. Most of them are considered again in the next section, which is directed toward probable causes of reactions. Even though they are grouped on the basis of simultaneous occurrence and/or apparent common etiology, the grouping should be regarded with some scepticism. Fever, for example, may occur for a variety of reasons – including the patient's underlying condition. Moreover, specific pharmacologic effects may share symptoms with anaphylaxis.

One of the most frequently noted types of reactions is that which appears pyrogenic in nature. The patient exhibits a rise in temperature, usually soon after the beginning of the infusion, and may also experience chills, shivering, and/or shaking. Despite this characteristic pattern, the actual aetiology is not easy to establish (Steere et al 1978, Quast et al 1981). Conversely, if the febrile response is not severe, the episode may not be reported. Thus the incidence of true pyrogenic reactions is nearly impossible to determine, inasmuch as both over-reporting and under-reporting can occur.

Vying with pyrogenic reactions for attention are those that appear to have an allergic basis. Urticaria is one of the most frequent symptoms. It may occur in the presence or the absence of more serious side effects, or may even precede them. Systemic reactions are sometimes called 'anaphylactoid,' a term that is broader than 'anaphylaxis' but carries fewer aetiologic implications. An anaphylactoid response may include dermatologic symptoms (urticaria and/or flushing), as well as blood pressure changes (usually hypotension), tachycardia, and respiratory symptoms such as chest tightness, shortness of breath, wheezing, or dyspnoea. The more serious reac-

Table 2.2   Types of untoward symptoms

1. Pyrogenic
   a. Fever
   b. Chills
   c. Shaking
2. Allergic, anaphylactoid
   a. Urticaria, flushing
   b. Hypotension
   c. Dyspnoea
   d. Tachycardia, palpitation
   e. Shock, anaphylaxis
3. Generalized reactions
   a. Nausea, vomiting
   b. Malaise
   c. Headache
   d. Injection site pain
4. 'Isolated' hypotension
5. Hypervolaemia, circulatory overload
6. Infectious disease
7. 'Chemical' changes

tions can present as shock; these may represent true anaphylaxis. A few cases of respiratory and/or cardiac arrest have been reported. These may be reversible by epinephrine, corticosteroids, etc. if the treatment is prompt enough (Ring et al 1979).

Sporadic reports deal with generalized, less serious symptoms such as gastrointestinal distress (nausea, vomiting), malaise, and headache. Whereas a non-specific symptom like pain at the injection site might reasonably initiate a search for a chemical aberration in the product, these others offer little help to the investigator seeking the cause or mechanism of the reaction. Moreover, specific pharmacologic agents can elicit symptoms that appear very non-specific.

One particular symptom, namely hypotension, is listed again, despite the fact that it was considered previously within the complex of allergic or anaphylactoid reactions. This is because hypotension is sometimes the only symptom reported; sometimes it occurs along with skin flushing. Typical of these 'isolated' hypotensive reactions were those elicited by PPF that contained prekallikrein activator (Alving et al 1978). As in the case of all symptoms, it is important to determine whether the hypotension is due to the albumin preparation, the patient's underlying condition, or the clinical procedure (e.g. haemodialysis) being performed.

A set of phenomena which is seldom found in lists of reported untoward reactions to albumin preparations is circulatory overload and its sequelae. Nonetheless, it has been described in the surgical literature (Weaver et al 1978, Dahn et al 1979) and bears mention here. That is, when patients who have been adequately resuscitated (hydrated) receive additional albumin solution, hypervolaemia can occur and detrimental pulmonary and/or cardiac effects can ensue.

Transmission of infectious disease by albumin preparations is an extremely rare event which has occurred only under 'extraordinary circumstances. Under such circumstances, both viral (Pattison et al 1976) and bacterial (Steere et al 1977) diseases have been transmitted. These are discussed later in an effort to relate the safety of albumin preparations to manufacturing characteristics noted above.

Changes detected by laboratory measurements (listed as 'chemical' changes for the sake of brevity) have been reported after the infusion of albumin preparations. These have sometimes, but not always, been accompanied by adverse clinical effects. They include metabolic alkalosis (Rahilly & Berl 1979), altered coagulation (Johnson et al 1979), hypernatraemia (Kalter & Reeves 1985), and accumulation of aluminum (Maher et al 1986). Their diversity alone suggests that, in many cases, these changes have gone unrecognized. Like circulatory overload, they serve to illustrate potential untoward effects that may occur in particular clinical settings or when several particular circumstances coincide.

CLASSES OF REACTIONS: PROBABLE (POSSIBLE) CAUSES

This section comprises a search for the causes of untoward reactions that have been observed and reported, as well as a brief examination of some potential sources of side effects. In the course of the former, many of the symptoms noted above are revisited. The approach, however, is not simply a step-by-step analysis of symptoms that have already been listed. Rather it represents an effort to classify, in a general way, the underlying causes themselves and to consider the resulting reactions within these classes. As noted in the foregoing section, some reactions can occur for more than one reason. Consequently, they may appear more than once in the following

Table 2.3 Classes of probable (possible) causes of reactions

1. The major protein
   a. Albumin
   b. Altered albumin
2. Additives
   a. Organic anions
   b. Sodium
3. Unintentional constituents (Class I)
   a. Contact activation factors
   b. IgA
   c. Metals
   d. Anions
4. Unintentional constituents (Class II)
   a. Bacteria
   b. Pyrogens
   c. Viruses
5. Unstandardized clinical uses
   a. Plasma exchange
   b. Inappropriate use
6. 'Different' uses

discussion. It is hoped that the value of this 'dual focus' will compensate for the redundancy it engenders.

Reactions to the major protein

The major protein in the preparations being considered is, of course, albumin. Accordingly, it should be the most likely suspect in the case of an untoward reaction. If, however, albumin is not altered during the manufacturing process (a supposition that admittedly is nearly impossible to prove – see Finlayson 1978), it should be a normal metabolite for the vast majority of recipients. One group in the apparently infinitesimal minority is composed of individuals who are homozygous for an albumin variant. Naylor et al (1982) have demonstrated antigenic differences between a genetic variant and 'normal' albumin. Nonetheless, even these authors concluded that the risk of developing antibodies against albumin is small and that the clinical significance of such antibodies is unknown.

Evidently then, if adverse clinical reactions to albumin molecules have an immunological basis, these molecules must have been altered in some way after they left the donor's circulation. The most readily detected changes that occur during manufacturing and storage of albumin preparations are increases in molecular size, i.e. the formation of high molecular weight aggregates.[*] It therefore does not seem surprising that patients who had undergone anaphylactoid reactions to albumin exhibited positive reactions to intradermal injection of aggregated albumin, lymphocyte transformation by aggregated albumin and/or precipitating antibodies to the 'macroaggregate' (Ring et al 1974, 1979). However, the investigators who made these observations concluded that the anaphylactoid reactions of these patients (each of whom had a history of allergy) were non-specific reactions to protein aggregates (Ring et al 1979).

There are additional examples of the difficulties encountered in establishing an allergic basis for reactions to albumin. Quast et al (1981) surveyed reactions reported over a 10 year period but gleaned no evidence that true allergic reactions occurred. Conversely, Paul et al (1981), whose patient clearly showed the symptoms of anaphylactic reaction – flushing, wheal formation, respiratory distress, and a similar response when albumin was given two days later – could detect no circulating antibodies to albumin. When Edelman et al (1985) used albumin for plasma exchange in a patient who had a previous anaphylactoid reaction to a different lot of albumin, no untoward signs appeared.

Untoward reactions to macromolecular aggregates of albumin need not be allergic in nature. Experimental studies have shown that these materials can produce reticuloendothelial blockade and thereby increase susceptibility

---

[*] This illustrates the inadequacy of the classification system. Inasmuch as these molecular aggregates (polymers) do not occur naturally, they could have been listed in either class of 'unintentional constituents.'

to shock (for summary, see Finlayson 1980). In view of the fact that more high molecular weight polymer is formed in the less purified albumin preparations, e.g. PPF (Yu & Finlayson 1984a), these products appear more likely to produce blockade than does purified albumin. Again, however, determining the extent to which this type of reaction occurs in the clinic is extremely difficult.

Reactions to additives

One additive that has already been mentioned is caprylate, which is used as a stabilizer. Although various adverse effects of caprylate have been demonstrated in experimental situations (for summary, see Yu & Finlayson 1984b), albumin was not involved in these experiments. Caprylate-stabilized albumin, on the other hand, was found to interfere with the blood grouping and typing of certain patients. Eventually, it was learned that the sera of these individuals contain fatty acid-dependent antibodies which, in the presence of caprylate, agglutinate all human erythrocytes in laboratory tests. This raised the possibility of caprylate-stabilized albumin preparations evoking erythrocyte clumping and attendant circulatory problems in vivo. When it was administered to a patient with fatty acid-dependent antibodies, albumin stabilized with caprylate produced no untoward reaction (Hossaini et al 1976). By contrast, some patients who had anaphylactoid reactions to human albumin showed positive skin reactions when caprylate-treated, non-aggregated (monomeric) albumin was injected intradermally (Ring et al 1979). Among these was one patient who exhibited no skin reaction to monomeric albumin alone.

Laboratory experiments in dogs revealed that acetate in PPF could lower the mean arterial pressure (Olinger et al 1979, Ng et al 1981). The frequency with which acetate actually caused hypotensive clinical reactions to PPF is unknown. An additional benefit of replacing the acetate with chloride, however, is illustrated by the observations of Rahilly & Berl (1979). These investigators found that when PPF containing a substantial quantity of acetate was used as the replacement fluid after thoracic-duct drainage, the patients developed metabolic alkalosis. In these cases, it was not only the additive, acetate, that was responsible for the untoward reactions, but also the relative absence of chloride. (In the US, formulation of albumin preparations is now done with sodium chloride; any acetate in the products is simply that remaining from fractionation buffers.)

A similar situation was revealed by the report of Kalter & Reeves (1985). Three critically ill cancer patients were given saline, a diuretic (furosemide), and albumin; all developed hypernatraemia. Although, as these authors pointed out, the role of albumin in this response is not clear, it emphasizes the need for clinicians to be aware of the non-protein constituents of albumin preparations and to consider their effects when a shift of body fluids is induced.

Reactions to unintentional constituents (Class I)

This section and the following one could easily have been grouped together. Certain reactions, however, have been placed in a separate category (Class II) because they were elicited by unintentional constituents which were present in the product because of a manufacturing discrepancy. The others (Class I) are discussed in the present section. Once again (see previous footnote), the classification is somewhat arbitrary. For example, in any retrospective examination, the manufacturing step at which pyrogens (Class II) entered a product is usually difficult to determine. Conversely, in some cases (Alving et al 1978, Milliner et al 1985a), steps responsible for the presence of Class I constituents have been identified.

Hypotensive and related reactions to partially purified albumin preparations had been reported sporadically for many years (for summary, see Finlayson 1980). It is now well established that many of these reactions were due to prekallikrein activator, which is also known as PKA, Hageman factor fragments, Factor XIIf, and β-XIIa (Alving et al 1978, van der Starre et al 1980, Heinonen et al 1982, van Rosevelt et al 1982). Because additional fractionation is employed in the purification process, prekallikrein activator is much less likely to occur in purified albumin than in PPF and similar products. Nonetheless, on occasion, it can be found in purified albumin as well (Alving et al 1978, Paton & Kerry 1981).

In view of these facts it is important for the user, as well as the manufacturer, of albumin preparations to have several considerations firmly in mind. First, prekallikrein activator acts by catalyzing the conversion of the recipient's prekallikrein to the active enzyme kallikrein. Kallikrein, in turn, acts on the patient's high molecular weight kininogen to release the potent vasodilator, bradykinin. This means that a small quantity of prekallikrein activator in the product administered can generate a large amount of bradykinin in the recipient. Second, under normal circumstances, bradykinin is rapidly inactivated in the body. Thus the amount of bradykinin present at any moment will be a function of the rate at which it is generated and the rate at which it is inactivated. This therefore means that the hypotensive effect of a product containing prekallikrein activator will depend on both the concentration of prekallikrein activator in the product and the *rate* at which the product is infused.

The industrial and clinical implications of the last sentence are obvious. It is necessary to know the prekallikrein activator content of the preparation being distributed and administered, or at least to know that it is below a certain defined level. Moreover, although patients on cardiopulmonary bypass are indeed vulnerable to the hypotensive effects of prekallikrein activator (inasmuch as the lung is a potent inactivator of bradykinin), this is by no means the only situation in which such reactions occur (Alving et al 1978, Heinonen et al 1982). Finally, the maximum permissible rate of administration of a particular preparation and its maximum allowable level of prekallikrein activator must be related to one another. For example, whereas a relatively higher concentration of prekallikrein activator may be tolerable in 20% or 25% albumin, whose viscosity and oncotic properties preclude overly rapid injection, that of 4% or 5% albumin, whose rate of infusion is unlimited, should be as low as possible.

Application of the foregoing information, as well as specific, quantitative tests for prekallikrein activator, has improved the safety of albumin products. Nevertheless, cases of 'isolated' hypotension continue to be reported. In some of these, it is difficult to determine whether the product or the clinical procedure was responsible. For example, albumin is sometimes used in conjunction with haemodialysis, but haemodialysis itself can produce hypotension. In other cases, there may be no obvious procedural cause of hypotension and the prekallikrein activator level may be very low. In some of these cases, the reactions may be caused by the presence of bradykinin itself in the product. In still others, the basis remains unknown. One possibility is the action of other contact activation factor(s), but the ultimate responsibility remains elusive. Presumably, kallikrein could evoke hypotension; however, it can be measured by simple modification of the methods for determining prekallikrein activator, and its heat lability makes it unlikely to occur in final albumin preparations in more than trace amounts. Whatever the exact cause(s), the greater probability of active contaminants in the less purified preparations and the rate-related nature of the reactions (see above) underline the appropriateness of caution. In the US, the labelling for PPF cautions against administration faster than 10 ml/min.

Of the proteins other than albumin, altered albumin, and contact activation factors present in albumin preparations, only IgA has been directly related to untoward reactions. PPF was found to elicit anaphylactic reactions in an IgA-deficient patient with circulating anti-IgA (Miller et al 1970).

Albumin is capable of binding many metal ions. One that has attracted considerable attention in recent years is aluminum. Although this element is usually excreted efficiently in the urine, patients with renal insufficiency and those who receive large amounts of aluminum parenterally are at risk of aluminum accumulation and toxicity. Symptoms of the latter can involve nervous tissue, the haemapoietic system, and bone (Sedman et al 1985). Sources of aluminum, in addition to food, include water used for dialysis, solutions for parenteral nutrition, and drugs used to combat hyperphosphataemia. Albumin preparations have now been added to this list (Milliner et al 1985b, Fell et al 1986, Maher et al 1986). Because, at present, albumin preparations are not routinely analyzed for aluminum content, clinicians whose patients receive large quantities of albumin products or receive them over an extended period of time and/or have compromised renal function should monitor these patients carefully and be aware of this potential source of aluminum loading.

It is not surprising that sensitive analyses can detect many metals in albumin preparations. Another metal that has been found in appreciable (and variable) quantities in albumin solutions is nickel (Leach & Sunderman 1985). As yet, no untoward reactions to albumin have been related to its nickel content. Nickel allergy, however, is relatively widespread. In view of the fact that severe allergic or anaphylactoid reactions can occur during (or after) intravenous infusions as a result of nickel sensitivity (Stoddart 1960), it appears possible that some reactions to albumin preparations may actually have been responses to small amounts of nickel.

The ability of albumin to bind anions is also well known. In addition to those already mentioned (chloride, caprylate, and endogenous long-chain fatty acids), lactate and citrate have been found associated with human albumin (Hanson & Ballard 1968). Most of the citrate apparently arises from the anticoagulant solution into which the blood was originally collected. Although the concentration of citrate in final albumin preparations is relatively low (Rahilly & Berl 1979, Chopek & McCullough 1980, Finlayson 1980), in some circumstances (e.g. plasma exchange in an infant) it might be sufficient to alter the patient's calcium balance.

Reactions to unintentional constituents (Class II)

Any occurrence of bacteria in the final container of an albumin preparation distributed for clinical use is a rare event. It represents an adverse breakthrough in the conflict between two continuously opposing forces. On the one hand are the many manufacturing steps designed to assure sterility. These include strict environmental control, careful preparation of the containers and closures, the membrane filtration itself, inspection of all vials of the product after an incubation period, and testing of representative samples for microbial growth. On the other hand are the ubiquity of microorganisms and the fact that preservatives are not used in the manufacturing process or in the final product. In view of the latter, the rarity of microbial contamination and its attendant clinical problems is truly remarkable because, despite all the manufacturing controls noted above, a low incidence of contamination could still escape detection. Steere et al (1977) described an episode of *Pseudomonas* bacteracmia caused by 25% albumin.

Viable bacteria need not be present in the final product to elicit an untoward reaction. If, at any stage of collection, storage, or manufacturing, bacteria should enter the material and produce endotoxin which is not removed at a later step in processing, the basis for a pyrogenic reaction will exist. Moreover, the bacteria themselves need never have been in contact with the plasma or the protein. Pyrogens, rather than the organisms, might have entered the process stream via raw materials, reagents, water, filters, or other equipment. As would be expected, this means that albumin preparations are much more likely to evoke a pyrogenic response than to cause microbial infection. For this reason, a series of controls similar to those listed in the previous paragraph have been instituted. Furthermore, the final product is tested for its ability to cause a febrile response in rabbits. Often, testing with Limulus amoebocyte lysate is also performed.

In spite of these precautions, serious difficulties confront the manufacturer. First, the Limulus test is very useful for detecting endotoxins, but interfering substances such as salts and protein may diminish its sensitivity. Thus calibration must be done with the individual albumin preparation being tested. Second, pyrogens other than endotoxins can produce febrile reactions. These can presumably be detected by the rabbit test, but they would escape notice in the Limulus assay. Finally, although these tests are very helpful, the quantitative relationships among the Limulus assay, the rabbit test, and human responses are not precise (Steere et al 1978). In addition, the dosage and clinical setting may have an important effect (see below).

Minimizing the frequency and severity of pyrogenic reactions requires participation of clinicians as well as manufacturers. The latter must be aware of the quality and the handling of the starting plasma. They can perform in-process monitoring with the Limulus test in addition to performing the other control activities already noted. Clinicians, for their part, must recognize the possibility of such reactions, record lot numbers of preparations administered, maintain constant surveillance, and promptly report and/or investigate untoward occurrences.

If bacterial infection is a rare side effect of albumin preparations, the incidence of viral infection must be near zero. The practice of heating for 10 hours at 60°C, which was initiated to inactivate hepatitis B virus, has been so effective that any exception must be considered to be a result of manufacturing failure. Such an event has been documented (Pattison et al 1976). Several lots of PPF made by a single manufacturer were responsible for an outbreak of hepatitis B, evidently as a result of inadequate heating. Although this unfortunate occurrence emphasizes the need for continuous attention to the heating step, its uniqueness illustrates the value of this step in eliminating danger from any other viruses (e.g. non-A, non-B hepatitis) that could be present.

Much current attention has been focused on the possibility of transmitting human T-lymphotropic virus type III/lymphadenopathy-associated virus by blood products. In view of the partitioning of this virus during fractionation (Wells et al 1986), its sensitivity to alcohol, even at low temperature (Wells et al 1986), and its extreme heat lability (Martin et al 1985), there is no risk of its transmission by albumin preparations manufactured as described in this chapter.

Unstandardized clinical uses

Thus far, the discussion of probable or possible causes of untoward reactions to albumin preparations has centred about the preparations themselves. In this section, attention is directed to clinical uses (specifically, those in which the appropriate regimen has not been defined or followed) and their possible role in adverse reactions.

Therapeutic plasma exchange is not a specific indication for albumin, at least in the US. Nevertheless, it enjoys fairly wide usage for this purpose, even though there have been few systematic studies and the optimal regimen is unknown (Chopek & McCullough 1980, Lasky et al 1984). Like other clinical manipulations, plasma exchange can be involved in the difficult situation of determining whether an untoward effect occurred as a result of the patient's underlying condition, the procedure itself, or the drug (in this case, the albumin preparation) administered. This important problem notwithstanding, it is worthwhile to consider certain aspects of the use of albumin solution as the replacement fluid.

The volume of replacement fluid employed in plasma exchange is large; for an adult patient it will usually be several litres. The rate of infusion is relatively high, hence the mechanisms for clearing any undesired components of the replacement fluid could be overwhelmed. If this is the case, levels of contaminants that might otherwise pass unnoticed could become clinically significant. Examples of this exist. In one study, plasma exchange produced a steep rise in the plasma aluminum concentration to a level that was of clinical concern, despite the facts that the albumin solution constituted less than one third of the total replacement fluid and the patient had stable renal function (Milliner et al 1985b). If the renal function had been compromised, continued accumulation of aluminum could have occurred (Maher et al 1986).

Fever and chills have been reported in patients undergoing plasma exchange with albumin as the replacement fluid. This suggests that pyrogenic reactions took place even though the products elicited no febrile response in the rabbit pyrogen test. In recent experiments (H. D. Hochstein, personal communication), albumin solution with a level of endotoxin that was undetectable by the standard rabbit pyrogen assay caused a continuous rise in temperature when administered to rabbits by sustained infusion.

A second category of clinical uses that deserve scrutiny comprises clinical settings in which guidelines for albumin use do exist. Often, it appears, these guidelines are ignored. In other cases, the clinical setting may be appropriate for albumin administration, but the actual use may not. Diffuse that this may be as a cause of untoward reactions, it is not a trivial consideration. Historically, albumin preparations have been over-used (Alexander et al 1979); indeed, their perceived safety may have contributed to use for non-indications. Although education and monitoring programmes can exert a significant corrective effect, a substantial proportion of patients continue to recieve albumin preparations inappropriately (Alexander et al 1982). Aside from the fact that misuse of these expensive products raises the cost of health care (Alexander et al 1979, 1982, Grundmann & Heistermann 1985), the inappropriately prescribed albumin may actually be detrimental to the patient. As noted previously, administration of supplemental albumin to patients who are already rehydrated can have negative effects on pulmonary (Weaver et al 1978), cardiac (Dahn et al 1979), and possibly, hemostatic (Johnson et al 1979) function. Moreover, as more is learned about pulmonary physiology and the chemical factors affecting capillary permeability in the lungs (Lancet Editorial 1986), clinical methods for assessing capillary leakage may be needed to guide albumin therapy. It is already obvious that administration of albumin to patients with inadequate alveolocapillary membrane integrity will not improve haemodynamic and pulmonary function, and may well worsen them (Shoemaker 1985).

'Different' clinical uses

This unusual category was created to accommodate possible causes of adverse reactions that did not reasonably fit under any other heading. The reasoning is as follows. Human albumin is employed for a variety of purposes other than plasma volume expansion. It is used to manufacture albumin microspheres and so-called 'soft' aggregates for radiolabelling and subsequent lung scanning. It is used as a stabilizer or carrier in certain intravenously administered protein products, and it serves a similar function in some that are injected by other routes. If, during the manufacturing of these products, new antigenic determinants were created on the albumin molecules, the patients receiving them might produce antibodies to these determinants. If these patients subsequently received conventional albumin preparations for plasma volume expansion, and the latter had been altered during processing in such a way as to be recognized by these antibodies, the basis for an allergic reaction could be established.

Such a possibility was considered when albumin microspheres first became available. Although anaphylactoid reactions to the aggregated albumin or microspheres themselves have been reported (Mather 1977), untoward effects resulting from cross-reaction with soluble albumin preparations have not been evident. On the other hand, two groups of investigators have concluded that β-propiolactone-modified human albumin is the allergen responsible for allergic reactions to a β-propiolactone-treated rabies vaccine (Baer et al 1985, Swanson et al 1985). It remains to be seen whether the antibodies involved recognize any form(s) of albumin in preparations for intravenous use. Brown et al (1985) examined the possibility of immunologic reactions to human albumin used as a stabilizer in allergen extracts; all test results were negative. Similarly, Grammer et al (1984, 1985) observed that although some haemodialysis patients had IgE antibodies against ethylene oxide-modified albumin, these antibodies did not react with the unmodified albumin preparation. This same group of workers, however, found that some of their patients with sensitivity to formaldehyde had IgE antibodies that reacted with both formaldehyde-albumin conjugates and albumin itself (Patterson et al 1986). Thus, even though this mechanism represents a rather unlikely basis for untoward reactions to intravenous albumin, it cannot be dismissed completely.

SOME GENERAL CONCLUSIONS

Compilations of untoward reactions to albumin preparations have repeatedly confirmed that the incidence of reported adverse reactions is low. As albumin preparations are put to new and different clinical uses, however, the true incidence of reactions – whether reported or not – may rise. One can then ask if it is possible to lower the absolute number of untoward episodes, given the fact that it is already quite low.

The first barrier to accomplishing this objective is the problem of recognition. This is doubly difficult inasmuch as the reactions are not only infrequent but also may fail to be clustered. To aid in this recognition, some of the major characteristics of the preparations and the reactions have been listed, as have probable and possible causes of adverse effects. (They have not been repeated here; the reader is referred to the lists themselves for a condensed overview.) The resulting pattern is a somewhat overlapping patchwork which may serve more as a guide to avoiding pitfalls than as a key to positive identification.

The difficulty of separating the influence of the patient's underlying condition and the clinical procedure from that of the albumin preparation itself has been emphasized repeatedly. Once this has been accomplished, still more work must be done to identify the specific cause of the reaction so as to provide a basis for avoiding it in the future. Suppose, for example, that the symptoms of a reaction which could reasonably be ascribed to albumin infusion were headache and hypotension. The alert investigator would realize that both of these symptoms can be elicited by bradykinin. Their occurrence in this particular case, however, might mean that the preparation contained bradykinin, that it contained an agent that released bradykinin (e.g. a catalyst or a precursor), that it contained some ingredient(s) which set off a chain of events that eventually culminated in the release of bradykinin, or that the reaction was evoked through a mechanism that did not involve bradykinin at all.

The inherent ambiguity is so great that it is probably wishful thinking to believe that the precise causes of all such reactions can be found. Nonetheless, it may be possible to diminish the number of untoward events if (1) albumin preparations are carefully monitored by manufacturers and regulatory agencies, with additional measurements incorporated into the quality control programme as their importance is recognized, (2) clinicians are aware of the contents – both intentional and unintentional – of these preparations and their potential impact on patients in various clinical conditions, (3) users recognize that the conditions of administration, such as the clinical setting and the rate of infusion, can influence the patient's response, and (4) albumin preparations are employed only when truly indicated.

REFERENCES

Alexander M R, Ambre J J, Liskow B I, Trost D C 1979 Therapeutic use of albumin. Journal of the American Medical Association 241: 2527–2529

Alexander M R, Alexander B, Mustion A L, Spector R, Wright C B 1982 Therapeutic use of albumin: 2. Journal of the American Medical Association 247: 831–833

Alving B M, Hojima Y, Pisano J J, et al 1978 Hypotension associated with prekallikrein activator (Hageman-factor fragments) in plasma protein fraction. New England Journal of Medicine 299: 66–70

Baer H, Anderson M C, Bernard K, Quinnan G 1985 Beta propiolactone treated human serum albumin (BPL-HSA) an allergen for humans receiving rabies vaccine. Journal of Allergy and Clinical Immunology 75:137

Barker L F 1976 Albumin products and the Bureau of Biologics. In: Sgouris J T, René A (eds) Proceedings of the Workshop on Albumin, DHEW Publication No. (NIH) 76–925. US Government Printing Office, Washington, pp 22–27

Brown J S, Ledoux R, Nelson H S 1985 An investigation of possible immunologic reactions to human serum albumin used as a stabilizer in allergy extracts. Journal of Allergy and Clinical Immunology 76: 808–812

Chopek M, McCullough J 1980 Protein and biochemical changes during plasma exchange. In: Berkman E M, Umlas J (eds) Therapeutic hemapheresis. American Association of Blood Banks, Washington, pp 13–52

Dahn M S, Lucas C E, Ledgerwood A M, Higgins R F 1979 Negative inotropic effect of albumin resuscitation for shock. Surgery 86: 235–241

Edelman B B, Straughn M A, Getz P, Schwartz E 1985 Uneventful plasma exchange with albumin replacement in a patient with a previous anaphylactoid reaction to albumin. Transfusion 25: 435–436

Fell G S, Shenkin A, Halls D J 1986 Aluminum contamination of intravenous pharmaceuticals, nutrients, and blood products. Lancet 1:380

Finlayson J S 1978 Assessment of changes that occur in proteins during fractionation. In: Sandberg H E (ed) Proceedings of the International Workshop on Technology for Protein Separation and Improvement of Blood Plasma Fractionation, DHEW Publication No. (NIH) 78–1422. US Government Printing Office, Washington, pp 542–555

Finlayson J S 1980 Albumin products. Seminars in Thrombosis and Hemostasis 6: 85–120

Grammer L C, Roberts M, Nicholls A J, Platts M M, Patterson R 1984 IgE against ethylene oxide-altered human serum albumin in patients who have had acute dialysis reactions. Journal of Allergy and Clinical Immunology 74: 544–546

Grammer L C, Shaughnessy M A, Paterson B F, Patterson R 1985 Characteristics of an antigen in acute anaphylactic dialysis reactions: Ethylene oxide-altered human serum albumin. Journal of Allergy and Clinical Immunology 76: 670–675

Grundmann R, Heistermann S 1985 Postoperative albumin infusion therapy based on colloid osmotic pressure. A prospectively randomized trial. Archives of Surgery 120: 911–915

Hanson R W, Ballard F J 1968 Citrate, pyruvate, and lactate contaminants of commercial serum albumin. Journal of Lipid Research 9: 667–668

Heinonen J, Peltola K, Himberg J-J, Suomela H 1982 Correlation of hypotensive effect of plasma protein fraction with plasma prekallikrein activator activity: A clinical study in patients having open-heart surgery. Annals of Thoracic Surgery 33: 244–249

Hossaini A A, Wasserman A J, Vennart G P 1976 Experimental induction of caprylate-dependent albumin antibodies. American Journal of Clinical Pathology 65: 513–517

Johnson S D, Lucas C E, Gerrick S J, Ledgerwood A M, Higgins R F 1979 Altered coagulation after albumin supplements for treatment of oligemic shock. Archives of Surgery 114: 379–383

Kalter S, Reeves W B 1985 Hypernatremia in cancer patients receiving normal saline, furosemide, and 'salt poor' albumin. Texas Medicine 81(12): 45–47

Lancet Editorial 1986 Adult respiratory distress syndrome. 1: 301–303

Lasky L C, Finnerty E P, Genis L, Polesky H F 1984 Protein and colloid osmotic pressure changes with albumin and/or saline replacement during plasma exchange. Transfusion 24: 256–259

Leach C N Jr, Sunderman F W Jr 1985 Nickel contamination of human serum albumin solutions. New England Journal of Medicine 313:1232

Maher E R, Brown E A, Curtis J R, Phillips M E, Sampson B 1986 Accumulation of aluminium in chronic renal failure due to administration of albumin replacement solutions. British Medical Journal 292:306

Martin L S, McDougal J S, Loskoski S L 1985 Disinfection and inactivation of the human T lymphotropic virus type III/lymphadenopathy-associated virus. Journal of Infectious Diseases 152: 400–403

Mather S J 1977 Adverse reaction to lung-scanning agent. Lancet 1: 907–908

Miller W V, Holland P V, Sugarbaker E, Strober W, Waldmann T A 1970 Anaphylactic reactions to IgA: A difficult transfusion problem. American Journal of Clinical Pathology 54: 618–621

Milliner D S, Feldman F, Shinaberger J H, Coburn J W 1985a Aluminum contamination of albumin-replacement solutions. New England Journal of Medicine 312:1390

Milliner D S, Shinaberger J H, Shuman P, Coburn J W 1985b Inadvertent aluminum administration during plasma exchange due to aluminum contamination of albumin-replacement solutions. New England Journal of Medicine 312: 165–167

Naylor D H, Anhorn C A, Laschinger C, Males F, Chodirker W B 1982 Antigenic differences between normal human albumin and a genetic variant. Transfusion 22: 128–133

Ng P K, Fournel M A, Lundblad J L 1981 Plasma protein fraction. Product improvement studies. Transfusion 21: 682–685

Olinger G N, Werner P H, Bonchek L I, Boerboom L E 1979 Vasodilator effects of the sodium acetate in pooled protein fraction. Annals of Surgery 190: 305–311

Paton C J, Kerry P J 1981 Prekallikrein activator in human albumin. Lancet 2:747

Patterson R, Pateras V, Grammer L C, Harris K E 1986 Human antibodies against formaldehyde-human serum albumin conjugates or human serum albumin in individuals exposed to formaldehyde. International Archives of Allergy and Applied Immunology 79: 53–59

Pattison C P, Klein C A, Leger R T, et al 1976 An outbreak of type B hepatitis associated with transfusion of plasma protein fraction. American Journal of Epidemiology 103: 399–407

Paul K, Schlesinger R G, Schanfield M S, Harbich J 1981 Reaction to albumin. Journal of the American Medical Association 245: 234–235

Quast U, Welge-Lüssen U, Sedlacek H H 1981 Adverse reactions in connection with albumin and other plasma substitutes. Developments in Biological Standardization 48: 131–142

Rahilly G T, Berl T 1979 Severe metabolic alkalosis caused by administration of plasma protein fraction in end-stage renal failure. New England Journal of Medicine 301: 824–826

Ring J, Messmer K 1977 Incidence and severity of anaphylactoid reactions to colloid volume substitutes. Lancet 1: 466–469

Ring J, Stephan W, Brendel W 1979 Anaphylactoid reactions to infusions of plasma protein and human serum albumin. Role of aggregated proteins and stabilizers added during production. Clinical Allergy 9: 89–97

Ring J, Seifert G, Lob G, Coulin K, Brendel W 1974 Humanalbuminunverträglichkeit: Klinische und immunologische Untersuchungen. Klinische Wochenschrift 52: 595–598

Sedman A B, Klein G L, Merritt R J, et al 1985 Evidence of aluminum loading in infants receiving intravenous therapy. New England Journal of Medicine 312: 1337–1343

Shoemaker W C 1985 Controversies in the pathophysiology and fluid management of postoperative adult respiratory distress syndrome. Surgical Clinics of North America 65: 931–963

Steere A C, Tenney J H, Mackel D C, et al 1977 Pseudomonas species bacteremia caused by contaminated normal human serum albumin. Journal of Infectious Diseases 135: 729–735

Steere A C, Rifaat M K, Seligmann E B Jr, et al 1978 Pyrogen reactions associated with the infusion of normal serum albumin (human). Transfusion 18: 102–107

Stoddart J C 1960 Nickel sensitivity as a cause of infusion reactions. Lancet 2: 741–742

Swanson M C, Rosanoff E, Gurwith M, Deitch M, Reed C E 1985 IgE and IgG antibodies to β-propiolactone associated with urticarial reactions to rabies vaccine. Annals of Allergy 55:295

van der Starre P, Sinclair D, Damen J, Brummelhuis H 1980 Inhibition of the hypotensive effect of plasma protein solutions by C_1 esterase inhibitor. Journal of Thoracic and Cardiovascular Surgery 79: 738–740

van Rosevelt R F, Bakker J C, Sinclair D M, Damen J, van Mourik J A 1982 Bradykinin-mediated hypotension after infusion of plasma-protein fraction. Journal of Laboratory and Clinical Medicine 100: 288–295

Weaver D W, Ledgerwood A M, Lucas C E, Higgins R, Bouwman D L, Johnson S D 1978 Pulmonary effects of albumin resuscitation for severe hypovolemic shock. Archives of Surgery 113: 387–392

Wells M A, Wittek A E, Epstein J S, et al 1986 Inactivation and partitioning of human T-cell lymphotropic virus, type III, during ethanol fractionation of plasma. Transfusion 26: 210–213

Yu M W, Finlayson J S 1984a Stabilization of human albumin by caprylate and acetyltryptophanate. Vox Sanguinis 47: 28–40

Yu M W, Finlayson J S 1984b Quantitative determination of the stabilizers octanoic acid and N-acetyl-DL-tryptophan in human albumin products. Journal of Pharmaceutical Sciences 73: 82–86

Computer applications to transfusion practice: principles and practice

INTRODUCTION

The management of a transfusion service requires all the skills needed to run a modern manufacturing and retailing business. Added to this is the vital fact that human lives are involved and therefore a high degree of technical and information accuracy is needed. It cannot be argued that safety should be achieved at any cost, but every attempt must be made to identify economic ways of achieving the greatest possible security in all procedures involved in the provision of products for patient care.

A major contribution to the high cost of safe procedures is the time required to carry out all the necessary or desirable checks and tests. It is not only the tests themselves that can be expensive, but the time taken to record and possibly look up further data. While it may not give complete control of costs, information management will provide not only cost benefits, but better data with which to run a transfusion service. It is fortunate, but not unexpected, that one of the main areas of computer development over the past decade has been in information processing. This covers the capture, storage and retrieval of data in an organized and efficient manner.

In order to establish the cost/benefit ratio of improvements which a computer system may bring to an organization, it is essential that management:
1. Understands the organisational function of the service.
2. Is aware of the capabilities of any computing system being proposed.
3. Has a clear set of objectives which the computer system will be required to meet.

Many organizations have developed computing systems without a clear idea of what they are trying to achieve. Many systems were brought in to handle accounts and payrolls. Any spare time was used to develop other functions and before long a state of chaos existed. Fortunately for the transfusion services in some countries there is no need to run payroll systems and the like, so the introduction of computing systems should not prove difficult, provided the above principles are noted.

Long before any computing development is undertaken in an organization, it is essential to establish clearly the aims and limitations of the proposed system. The 'Grand Plan' should not be implemented unless funds, staff and time are available and it can be projected that it will be cost effective.

The transfusion service is a complex organization. It is a rare, though not unique branch of a health care service which produces a therapeutic material for patient use. It must therefore carefully control its supply of raw material and its subsequent processing. It must also maintain accurate records of all the recipients of these products over a long period of time. This is especially important as the service becomes more developed and treatments more sophisticated.

ESSENTIAL ASPECTS OF A COMPUTING SYSTEM IN A TRANSFUSION SERVICE SETTING

The essential aspects of a good computing system can be summarised as follows:

Reliability

Any person wanting (and permitted) to use the system must find it accessible and the data accurate. Not all the data need be available at the press of a button, but in some areas, for example a blood bank where blood and blood products are issued to wards and operating theatres, the system, and hence the data, must be available at all times. In other areas an immediate response will not be so vital, for example the data required for blood donor call-up.

System response times are often given such a high priority that the reliability of the data is overlooked. It must not be forgotten that the data is the most important and valuable element of the whole system. Thus accurate data is essential and accuracy is reflected, not only in its contents, i.e. characters and numbers, but in its structure and how that structure reflects the 'world' it is intended to represent.

Good design

Good design is partially reflected in the content and structure of the data which is expected to describe the system being computerized. It requires an in-depth understanding of how the service functions and in what areas it is likely to develop and expand. Good quality management information can only be obtained with the use of consistent data which is checked and verified repeatedly. This checking and verification should be fully automatic and not require the user to perform any 'extra' tasks.

The functions that the system is to perform must be easy to understand

and use. Ideally these functions should reflect transfusion centre current practice and not require a vast amount of re-training. There may however be areas where change is necessary and it is here that education has an important role to play.

The system must be designed to have good recovery procedures not only from the occasional data input error, but from total power or systems failure. This requires a high degree of discipline in backup procedures especially in such areas as the blood bank where there is a need for a system which runs 24 hours a day. All too frequently systems are designed which fail to appreciate the danger of losing a large quantity of data should the machine fail.

Cost effective

This is probably one of the most frequently used phrases when computing systems are being discussed. It is one of the most difficult things to predict and measure, but this should not rule out attempts to quantify the definite, likely and possible benefits that may be derived from a computing system.

The easiest items to quantify are the hardware and software and possibly its long term maintainance. An item hardly ever taken into consideration is the long term replacement of the equipment, especially when it has been running for several years and there is a vast quantity of data to be retained and therefore transferred to replacement equipment. This problem can be overcome by giving careful consideration to the software environment of the data and attempting to ensure that similar environments are specified for replacement hardware. Software standards play an important part in ensuring success in this area. Thus if the system has been developed using internationally recognized languages and data base standards, then the transfer of the developed system and data to a manufacturer's new machine will prove to be comparatively easy. This is also important if the user wishes to transfer the system onto a different manufacturer's hardware, provided it has these standard languages and data base systems.

The most difficult item of expenditure to estimate is the development time of the system. To some extent the more detailed the design study is, the more the problems should be understood and therefore the easier the development should be. It should be emphasized that on many occasions this is not the case as some problems only become apparent when a system is partially developed and being test run. Also the rate at which different groups within the transfusion centre complete tasks may severely restrict the overall pace of the development. While there must be some management control of these projects, the amount of management time should not need to be excessive. A small dynamic team will nearly always outperform the large management-dependant group, provided the task is not too large and the individual members of each team understand the nature of the problems they have to resolve.

On the benefits side of the cost-effective equation, the most important item, often difficult to quantify, is an improved use of resources both human and material. This is especially important in the community based transfusion service where we depend on donors to give their blood freely and they therefore demand that we treat them with due consideration and use their gift to the best advantage of all. It may not always be possible to reduce the number of staff involved in such activities as the care and selection of donors and the supervision of blood withdrawal, but it is essential that the staff involved derive a high degree of personal satisfaction from using the computer system and that this results in their ability to provide a superior (more personalized) service. This can be achieved, particularly if they are involved at the earliest stages of the computer system development. Imposition of computing systems on staff, without their involvement in the development, can lead to difficulties during implementation.

The less obvious items of expenditure in the system, and often forgotten, are the consumables. These range from printer ribbons through bar-coded labels to magnetic tapes and disks. These must be included in the cost equation as they will continue for the length of the systems lifetime.

AREAS OF APPLICATION

A transfusion service may usefully be sub-divided operationally into three main activities areas as shown in Figure 3.1.

Although the system is linear in that one area feeds into the other, there is a feedback loop which may be used to regulate the total system, see Figure 3.2.

The main controlling factor for this feedback should be the demands clinical users place on the transfusion service through its blood bank. Whilst the provision of blood and blood products depends almost totally on the supply available from donors, the supply of fractionated plasma products will almost certainly depend upon an external source which may be commercial or otherwise. If the transfusion centre is involved with the

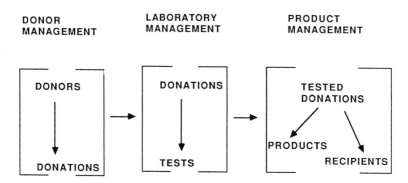

Fig. 3.1 Main activity areas of transfusion service.

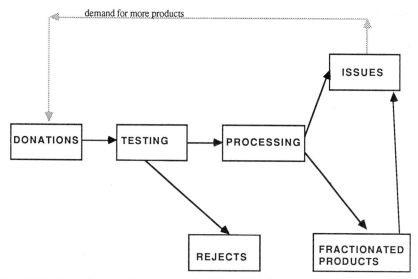

Fig. 3.2 Feedback loop regulating transfusion service activities.

supply of material for subsequent plasma fractionation, then this will require careful computer management planning as the derived products may take several weeks/months to produce and it is essential that full tracking facilities are available from patient to donor.

For the system to work smoothly it is necessary to determine how quickly the supply end of the system, donor call-ups, need to respond to sudden increases in demands. This must play an important role in the management of donor computer systems. A sluggish response will require the blood bank to hold large buffer stocks and possibly lead to wastage, whereas a rapid response time will enable the blood bank to cover its needs with lower stock levels and hopefully better utilization of stocks.

From a computing aspect, the management of donors and call-ups is a standard data processing task. Given the correct data it should be possible to call up any selection of donors at any time to meet an emergency. However, it is important not to reduce the reserve capacity of the donor pool to such an extent that it jeopardises future emergency demands.

The function of the laboratories in the system is to provide diagnostic and quality assurance facilities in an efficient and safe manner. Recent developments have greatly helped to achieve this goal more easily: these include, for instance, automated systems for generating and capturing data from blood grouping instruments and the use of bar-coded labels. Because of the high level of technology used in this area (blood grouping) it is most important that a comprehensive backup facility is carefully developed in order to avoid major problems when the automated testing system fails.

As more tests are introduced, for example HIV antibody testing, systems should be so designed so that the data can be incorporated into the system without the need for major redesign, which is expensive and frustrating to laboratory workers who are downstream of the new technology.

In all these laboratory based tests a most important aspect to be born in mind is that of 'sample identification' (ID). To operate any test procedure without good sample ID, will reduce the validity of the data generated and possibly eliminate the high degree of security offered by the more automated systems.

As has already been stated, the blood bank plays an important role in the feedback loop. Because of this it is important that the data generated in these areas are highly accurate and continually monitored. By the very nature of this aspect of a transfusion medicine service, it is also vital that the system be as robust as possible while at the same time capable of responding quickly to urgent requests. The development of a good blood banking computer system is a complex exercise and requires a clear understanding of the needs and methods used by the staff (laboratory and clinical) who are responsible for it.

Other areas that may be addressed in transfusion centres include:
Ante-natal testing
Tissue typing
Administration
Research and development

DEVELOPING A STRATEGY

Once it has been decided to introduce a computer system into a transfusion centre, a development strategy must be quickly established. Since the system being computerized is linear, it is possible to begin developing the system in any area and eventually complete the loop. In fact this is not always practicable. We may consider each starting point in turn and indicate the various pro's and con's.

Donor management

The major advantage of beginning to develop a transfusion centres totally integrated computer system from this area is that the donor record is a core item of data. Without the donor we have no donations and hence no service. To each donor identification record we may attach various items of data such as individual donations, test results, derived products and recipients. This structure is illustrated in Figure 3.3.

Because the donor is such an important 'data item', it is possible to develop a totally wrong model of the computer system if a careful data analysis and system design is not carried out. This process takes time and requires a great amount of patience from donor management and laboratory staff who will be eager to progress rapidly to system implementation. Implementation requires a large quantity of data to be in place before the

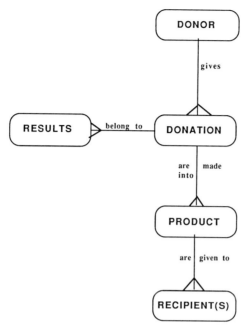

Fig. 3.3 Data associated with donation record.

system can begin to provide suitable data for the laboratory staff in particular. It is essential, therefore, to avoid a situation in which staff have to operate two different systems, one fully computerized and the other not. This leads to errors, frustration and possibly significant staff resistance to any further computerization.

Laboratory system

The temptation to begin developing computer systems in the laboratory is difficult to resist. This is especially so with the availability of many different sophisticated pieces of equipment which can be so easily linked to any computer. However, it is important to recognize that if the laboratory area is addressed first, it is possible that the overall centre plan/strategy may become distorted and the donor becomes an irritating adjunct to a grandiose and dominating laboratory system.

It can however, be argued that a sensible start may be made in the laboratory without involvement of donor data, provided it is done by the careful use of single microprocessors. Single microprocessors can be used to extend the effectiveness of the automated equipment well beyond the original scope envisaged by the manufacturer, but at the same time still acting as data capture devices. These microprocessor systems can become important items in the overall centre plan as they can eventually be used as backup should the main system fail. Because of their low cost and provided they have good software, it is possible to develop a pilot system in an interactive manner with the staff involved. Such a development may provide a good development environment and an understanding between laboratory and computer staff. From these interactions many of the operational problems will emerge and resolutions found which, provided there is effective management, have a profoundly beneficial effect on the overall centre system development.

Blood bank

It is extremely difficult to begin the development of an integrated system in this area. It is by nature a busy place involving testing and issuing of blood/products for individual patients and staff will not have the time to input the necessary data to run the system. They may also be prone to error if a high volume of manual input is required.

Logically a clinically interfaced blood banking system should be closely connected to the laboratory system, whether the data comes from the main machine or a microprocessor. If a well defined interface between the laboratory system and the blood bank system is specified, then it is possible to develop both in parallel. It must be remembered, however, that not all the products handled in the blood bank will necessarily originate in the transfusion centre, since fractionated plasma products may be imported from an external fractionation centre.

Once staff begin to operate a blood bank system they will quickly become dependent on it. This makes any further developments difficult and therefore makes it difficult to withdraw facilities for major modifications.

Main frame or microprocessors

Another strategy aspect to be considered when introducing computerization to the transfusion centre is whether to start the development on microprocessors or to begin on a 'Main Frame' type mini. With the greatly improved cost/perfomance of modern mini computers, it is possible to begin development on such machines from the start.

It may be argued that there are several important advantages to be gained if development is begun on a series of microprocessors. The most obvious one is that they will form an essential part of the back-up facilities should the larger system fail. For this reason it is important to ensure that the development path of the micros fits in with the philosophy of the larger systems. Another important factor in this micros type of development is that a gradual build up of expertise among the computer and laboratory staff is developed. This is extremely important for the transfusion centre as a whole as it contributes to a high level of confidence in the computer systems that are being developed, and should be a useful opportunity for laboratory staff to question the necessity and validity of work they undertake.

The limited capabilities of micros may, however, force the centre development team to limit their objectives. Provided the limitations are within a reasonable time period it is possible that more realistic goals can be established and achieved. Because of the low cost of micros, it is easier to 'pilot' systems in different areas of the service, thereby facilitating transfer to a main frame system.

The main limiting factor in the use of microprocessors for the whole centre system is one of data storage. A typical transfusion centre handling 50–100 000 donations per year may require an organized storage space of about 100 megabytes (a megabyte is approximately 1 million characters). This does not include the needs of antenatal testing, tissue typing, administration and research and development. While storage devices of 100 megabytes may be addressed on micros, the management of the data is often difficult and frequently not cost effective. Another drawback to the continued use of micros for the total syetem is the inability for different processes to 'share' data. Local Area Networks (LAN's) have tried to address this problem, but very few have really succeeded. The main problem with the LAN is not so much the access to the data, but the control over access to it and the need to preserve its structure and confidentiality.

The main advantages of developing the system on a mini are that such machines have a large storage capacity and powerful software with which to manipulate it. It should be noted however that the selection of the software is extremely important. Its quality may well determine how quickly the system can be developed and how easy it is to document.

Any large computing system will require maintenance, even if it is only to install the vendor's new releases of the software. From the transfusion service point of view the greatest risk posed by the the single mini is the problem of backup. A second large machine may be ideal, but the cost will almost certainly rule it out. For this reason alone, to develop parts of the system initially on micros and move the applications onto a larger system at a later date may be the best strategy for computerizing in a transfusion centre.

Provision of working standards

No matter which approach is chosen for the task, it is essential that a set of standards for system development are established. The main areas to be covered by these standards are:

Programme specifications

No programme should ever be developed without a specification as to what it is intended to do. Without this, one cannot determine if the programme has met its objectives. Even a few sentences may suffice so that the implementation team has an end objective and the user knows what he/she is being given.

System specifications

This information will be essential for anyone required to maintain or modify the software at a later date. It must define clearly how the software operates and what items of data it manipulates. For large data base applications, this information enables the team to modify programmes and predict accurately the effect these will have on the total system. It is also required to pinpoint areas that will require amendments should the underlying software be altered by the vendor.

User guides

These are an essential requirement if the users are to maximize the use of the system. Ideally these documents should be written jointly by both the person who developed and implemented the system and the people who intend to use it. This should ensure that both parties use terms that are fully understood and explained.

AN EXAMPLE

In order to try and put the principles described into perspective, it may be helpful to describe the development of an actual system currently established in the South East Scotland Transfusion Service and its development from 1980 to the present day.

This transfusion centre covers an area with a population of 1.25 million people. It collects 80 000 units of blood annually from a donor panel of approximately 100 000. It is unusual in that it also operates a full cross-matching service for most of the hospitals in the city of Edinburgh. This requires about 30 000 compatibility tests a year. As a result of this, the 'feed-back' loop mentioned earlier needs to operate very effectively, since the supply and demand areas are within the same organization.

In 1980 the author was invited to look at the centre's operation and develop a strategy for full computerization. At this time two major factors influenced the development path chosen: that it would take at least three years to obtain approval for major computer funding and that there was an immediate need to relieve the high clerical load in the donor management office.

Both these factors led to a development path starting with microprocessors and eventually leading to a 'Main Frame' system. The first objective was to attend to the donor office problem and at the same time ensure that the system would not hinder future, and at that time undefined, plans. A simple data base system running on a Cromemco System 3 was selected and a suite of basic programmes developed to enable donor call-ups to be run.

What evolved was in fact an 'addressograph' system, but with the benefit of being a data capture mechanism for the larger system. However, in addition to solving a specific problem, this donor call-up system helped to illustrate the relationship between donor, donations and recipients. It was an ideal way to begin to understand the organization of the transfusion service. The total capital cost for this development was less than £10 000.

The next phase of the development was to continue the deployment of microprocessors, and at the same time establish the operational requirements for the larger system. This information was necessary for the estimation of the capital and revenue funds required.

The donor grouping laboratory was chosen for the next stage of the development. This choice was again dictated by circumstances: the imminent introduction of bar-coded labels and the need for a modified checking procedure and as a necessary first step towards the development of a clinically based blood banking system.

It was decided that the blood banking system should run on a different processor in order to improve the overall reliability of the system. It was also intended that the system developed would be able to operate in peripheral (local hospital) blood banks, thus ensuring a uniform high quality of data throughout the region.

A major part of the implementation philosophy for the micro based systems was the use of the UCSD(p) operating system (1) and the Pascal programming language (2). The UCSD(p) operating system was chosen for its ease of use and portability over several machines. This operating system is also available in a multi-user form and thus proved ideal for the clincial blood banking system.

Pascal was chosen because it was a high level structured language and internationally agreed standards exist. This provides a development path onto many other micro and mini machines, should the requirement arise. There are at present many other different languages and systems used within laboratory computing, the best known ones include MUMPS, Pick and Unix. However, at the time when the transfusion centre development began none of these systems were yet available on the range of micros the centre could afford. Moreover, the author already was quite familiar with Pascal and the UCSD(p) systems and, as a result, more time could be given to solving the problems in hand rather than learning new languages and operating systems.

The specification for the donor grouping system read as follows.

COMPUTERIZED PACK LABELLING SYSTEM
PRELIMINARY SPECIFICATION

The aim of this specification is to define a system which will be made up of several independent components run on a microprocessor on its own. The functions carried out in this area are time critical in that it is desirable to make blood/products available to the blood bank as soon as possible. In view of this it is essential that:

1. The system does not become an integral component in the blood bank area until it is thoroughly tested.

2. The amount of time required to run the system does not involve an increase in the work load in the blood bank area.

The long term aims have been to develop a computer system which is robust and at the same time may act as a backup for any future main frame system. It is intended that bar-code readers will play an important part in the data capture procedures, hence it is vital that we recognize the areas where international standards apply.

The system was developed on the Sirius microprocessor using the UCSD(p) operating system. This enabled it to be easily transferred to other UCSD(p) systems. The major functions of the system were defined as follows:

1. To enable blood and its products to be labelled and verified using bar-coded labels and bar-code readers.

2. To begin to automate the collection of data for all blood and products handled in the donor grouping area.

Initially the donor grouping system, later called the PLV (Pack Labelling/Verification system) was based on a totally manual input system. Bar codes were used with readers to speed the input and verification of the data. Once the data was in the system, a standard pack verification module could be used to complete the process. An immediate spin-off from this system was the ease with which the workload statistics for this area were collected and available for analysis.

The donor grouping system was introduced into routine service in mid 1983, initially using one machine, but very quickly requiring two. Once established, the interface to the blood banking system was defined and developed.

In December 1983 a Kontron G2000 was delivered to the transfusion centre. Because of the way the Pack Labelling/Verification (PLV) system had been designed, only the data capture module had to be slightly modified in order to accept data from the Kontron machine. As a safeguard the manual input process was not eliminated, in case the Kontron system failed and manual techniques had to be used. As an example of the modularity of this software, the Kontron input module has been replaced by a module for accepting data from a locally developed micro-plate blood grouping system. This particular micro-plate version is now in regular use in three Scottish transfusion centres. This enables these centres to use the clinical blood bank system (developed in the Edinburgh Centre) which has a standard interface to the PLV system.

In August 1983 funding for a Mini was agreed and the tendering process begun. It was now that the system requirements were translated into operational requirements against which competing manufacturers could quote. In May 1984 a Data General MV4000 was installed with the following major software components:

1. A data base system.

2. A transaction processing system.

3. An ANSI standard Cobol system.

A major consideration for this choice of machine was the fact that the software adhered to internationally defined standards. The machine is one of the modern 32 bit virtual addressing systems which makes it ideal for a multi-user data base environment.

As with the initial micro development, the first area to be developed on the mini system was the Donor Management module. The aim was to produce a system which, to the user, closely resembled the micro based system, thus maintaining the users confidence and at the same time allowing the micro based system to be phased out without difficulty. It was recognized that the micro system, unlike the PLV micro system, would not be able to provide the Donor management system with a backup. This was considered to be acceptable since the workflow in the donor office was such as to permit a period of machine 'down time' in hours.

By May 1985 (12 months after the delivery of the mini) a totally integrated data base had been defined for the centre an initial set of programs to handle most of the donor management requirements was ready. The data from the microprocessors was transferred into the MV4000 as the various donor panels were called up. This phasing enabled the staff to become familiar with the new system. The most immediate advantage of the new (mini) system was the fact that the data is held in a common file and is therefore accessible from several different terminals concurrently. By January 1986 about 80 000 donors were being held on the system and user acceptance was high.

Probably the most important development of the total system has been that associated with the multi-user clinical blood banking system. Some preliminary development, using the UCSD(p) operating system and Pascal Programming language had already been carried out but this project proved to be a good example of one in which the initial concepts were right, but implementation and installation were difficult.

The most difficult aspect of the clinical blood banking development was how to test and introduce the system into a working area which provides a 24 h emergency service and where time for training and testing is restricted. Moreover because of staff rotations during the night and at weekends, the number of staff requiring training is high, and indeed, involved 40 people. As a result of these difficulties a strategy was evolved in which the system was introduced in a phased way using a series of modules, commencement focused on non-critical areas with a gradual expansion into others as confidence grew and the phased programme was led by a designated member of the blood banking technical staff who was attached to the computer development team not only to act as a trainer but also to channel back problems and innovations to the computer development team.

The basic specification for the clinical blood banking system read as follows:

1. To set up an inventory system to record the 'receipt/issue/return' of blood/products to the blood bank. An up-to-date status of the blood bank will be provided as a result of all transactions.

2. To accumulate a file of recipients (actual and potential) who have identified red cell membrane antibodies.
3. To identify requests for crossmatches and group, save and screens and to record the outcome of these procedures.

The first phase of the clinical blood banking system was put into operation in March 1985. It was based on a Sage IV multi-user microprocessor using the UCSD(p) system. It provided access for five terminals, one of which was able to control two processes. Since the PLV system was by now in routine use, the direct input of all labelled blood/products was carried out using a simple record transfer technique. Each record held all the relevant details for a single product, which included product type, blood group, expiry date and any known phenotype information. There were some initial system software problems as well as the expected application software problems.

Initially only two functions were run on the system, namely: the issue and return of 'bulk issues' to peripheral hospital blood banks; the collection of data concerning patients with cross-matching problems. These areas were deliberately selected for the first phase of the project because they were not time-critical and thus enabled the blood bank staff to become familiar with the keyboards etc. As confidence grew, the system was further expanded to cover crossmatching requests for selected hospitals and eventually by July 1985, all blood banking areas served by the Transfusion Centre.

By the Autumn of 1985 it became apparent that the system had high user acceptance, to the extent that it was becoming overloaded. On a typical day 100 cross-match requests were input along with 300–400 new unit movements. (A unit movement has been defined as the issue/return of a unit). At peak periods, the system was having to process over 200 transactions/hour. While this is a very small number for a main frame, it led, during these peak periods, to prolonged response times on the micro system. The main reason for this was not the processor, but the access times to the disk. This also meant that it was not possible to run any analysis programmes during the day as these would also slow down the routine system.

Another important feature of the clinical blood banking system, which only became apparent with its use, was the speed with which data could be input. This was due to the use of bar-coded labels and wand readers. The bar-coded labels were used both on the blood products and on the request forms. The only time that a user was therefore required to input data by hand was when a potential recipient was initially registered. Once they had been registered and allocated their unique bar-coded identifier, all the relevant data could be retrieved by the wanding of their bar coded I.D. This facility led to data input rates many times faster than normal handtyped input and consequently the system response appeared to be relatively slow.

In Spring 1986 the original Sage IV was replaced by a Stride 440 which had a faster processor and a much faster disk. The transfer of both the data and the programmes to this new micro system was carried out in less than an hour, only marginally longer than the standard back-up time. This was wholly due to the complete portability of the code and data within the UCSD(p) system. The subsequent response times have proved to be excellent, permitting two extra terminals to be added and additional features introduced. For instance, the system has been extended to handle all plasma fractionated products (factor VIII, albumin etc.) issues.

The release of the Sage IV in favour of the Stride 440 has provided a back-up machine and also enables the staff to carry out many different analyses of the data being generated. These include blood and blood product usage figures for different hospitals and even at ward level. These blood/blood product figures give a graphic illustration of certain aspects of clinical performance which are likely to be of value in the context of clinical audit. The system also enables the transfusion centre to examine its workload, over 24 hour/7 day week periods and provides ready information on the length of time that units of blood or blood products are out of the blood bank. This latter feature is particularly important if one is to permit the re-issue of units that have been returned from hospital wards or even peripheral (hospital) blood banks.

Since every movement of a blood product is recorded by the clinical blood banking system, it is possible to provide a complete individual unit history for every product lodged into the blood bank. This includes a product that is never cross-matched, but is issued for further processing when it becomes time expired. As well as unit histories, the system can also provide patient histories. These include a record of every transfusion request, the number of units and products involved and the final outcome for each episode.

The next phase of the overall centre development is to move the PLV system onto the main-frame machine and then develop a long term file storage system for the data generated by the clinical blood banking system. In view of the comparative cheapness of the Stride machine, it is considered feasible to have a complete backup machine available. This machine can be used to analyse the blood bank data and also for any further developments. Because of the well-defined interface to the PLV system, it will require very little effort to link the Stride to the MV4000 mini main-frame unit.

The most important benefit from the whole development in the transfusion centre to date is the improvement in the quality of the data in all areas and the confidence the staff have gained in the computer system. Management now has accurate data upon which sound decisions may be based. At the same time a backup system exists for every area so far covered. Because of their constant involvement with the development of the system, the level of user satisfaction is high.

TOMORROW

As microprocessors become more powerful, it is inevitable that some functions can be taken away from the large (mini) systems. The main future use of the main frame is likely to be the storage of large quantities of data in an organized manner. It is from this long term data that we can provide complete and accurate records of every donation, test and transfusion event. At present a file store of 700 megabytes is available to the Edinburgh Centre. In 10 years time this may well have to be increased at least ten fold.

Another area for future development is in data capture. The cost-effectiveness of issuing donors with plastic registration cards with magnetic strips is not far away. Used in conjunction with new portable microprocessors, data capture at donor (bleeding) session will be made extremely easy and accurate. At the other end of the transfusion chain, improved methods of patient and sample identification will make it possible to almost eliminate the problem of transfusing patients with incompatible blood due to clerical error. In order to achieve this goal, it will be helpful to link the transfusion centre's system with the hospitals' own computing systems. Such developments will be difficult and required thorough forward planning if they are to be genuinely effective and user acceptable.

REFERENCES

Jensen K, Niklaus W, Pascal 1974 User Manual and Report. Springer-Verlag
UCSD p-System and UCSD Pascal 1981 Version IV.∅. 2nd Edition. SofTech Microsystems

Transfusion and neonatal intracranial haemorrhage

INTRODUCTION

Intraventricular haemorrhage is the most common neurological condition occurring in pre-term infants (Alan & Volpe 1986, Volpe 1981a). The association between intraventricular haemorrhage and very low birth weight was first noted in 1919 by Ylppö (1919) although the problem of intracranial haemorrhage associated with birth trauma subsequently occupied the minds of researchers in the 1930s and 40s. It was not until the publication of data from the British National Birthday Trust Perinatal Mortality Survey of 1958 that the frequency of intraventricular haemorrhage by birthweight and gestation was first documented (Fedrick & Butler 1970); it is now recognized that the incidence of intraventricular haemorrhage is of the order of 30–40% in infants weighing < 1500 g (Beverley et al 1984a, Cooke 1981, Tarby & Volpe 1982) and its prevention is one of the major challenges facing neonatologists. Other forms of intracranial haemorrhage are now uncommon and rarely occur in the neonatal population.

It has been claimed that transfusion may play a key role in the prevention and management of intraventricular haemorrhage in neonates weighing < 1500 g.

ANATOMICAL CONSIDERATIONS

Approximately 80–90% of intraventricular haemorrhages originate in the germinal matrix at the head of the caudate nucleus and the foramen of Munro (Hambleton & Wigglesworth 1976, Grunewald 1951). However, the site of origin is related to gestational age so that in pre-term infants the majority of bleeds occur over the caudate nucleus (Hambleton & Wigglesworth 1976) whilst in term infants the site is predominantly from the choroid plexus (Donat et al 1978). This site in premature infants is related to the presence of the germinal matrix which consists of an immature vascular rete which is devoid of supportive mesenchymal elements (Pape & Wigglesworth 1979a). As a consequence, the capillaries are extremely fragile and prone to rupture; with increasing maturity the germinal matrix regresses so that by term it is dissipated (Yakovlev & Rosales 1970). The incidence of intraventricular haemorrhage can be directly related to the presence of this germinal matrix.

AETIOLOGY

Many factors have been associated with the development of intraventricular haemorrhage, some of which are respiratory distress syndrome and its associated blood gas abnormalities (Levine et al 1982, Fujimura et al 1979, Kenny et al 1978), pneumothorax (Lipscomb et al 1981, Hill et al 1982), birth asphyxia (Beverley et al 1984b), mode and place of delivery (Beverley et al 1984a, Clark et al 1981), rapid infusion of hyperosmolar fluids (Papile et al 1978a), patent ductus arteriosus (Beverley et al 1984a) and many more. All these factors probably exert their effect via the cerebral circulation where it is known that vascular autoregulation is impaired (Lou et al 1979a), this being particularly so after an asphyxial insult (Lou et al 1979b). As a consequence, the cerebral circulation is pressure passive leading to large changes in cerebral blood flow with changes in blood pressure. The fragile capillary network in the germinal matrix is thus at particular risk of rupture when changes in blood pressure occur; these haemodynamic changes have recently been documented by Perlman et al (1983) who were able to look at blood flow in the anterior cerebral artery and relate this to systemic blood pressure. They noticed that only 2 of 23 infants with a stable systemic arterial blood pressure developed intraventricular haemorrhage compared with 20 of 27 infants who had unstable blood pressures, so confirming the importance of haemodynamic changes.

Coagulation factors

With the rupture of the capillaries in the germinal matrix the size of the subsequent haemorrhage will, in part, be determined by the efficiency of the neonate's haemostatic system. It is known that in the region of the germinal matrix there is excessive fibrinolytic activity (Giles et al 1971) so it is of paramount importance to the infant to have effective haemostasis to limit the size of haemorrhage. The remainder of this chapter will review the history of coagulation disorders in relationship to the development of intraventricular haemorrhage for it is in this area that transfusion medicine may or may not have a rôle to play.

The development of the neonatal haemostatic system

Normal haemostasis is a function of the interaction between blood vessels, platelets, coagulation proteins, anti-coagulants and fibrinolysis. As already described the capillaries and blood vessels in the pre-term infant are more fragile than those in the term infant. It is known that platelet counts are within the normal adult range in pre-term infants but it would appear that platelet function is impaired when compared to the full term infant (Stuart 1979). As far as the clotting factors are concerned, fibrinogen, factor V, VIII and XII are essentially normal in pre-term infants, though fibrinogen may not be as functionally active. The vitamin K dependant factors II, VII, IX and X and the contact factors XI, XII, prekallikrein and high molecular weight kinogen are reduced to 20–30% in pre-term and 50% in term infants when compared with adults (Beverley et al 1984c, Buchanan 1986). The anticoagulants alpha 2 macroglobulin, antithrombin III, protein C and protein S are either functionally reduced or reduced in total activity, thus there is a theoretical risk that in the presence of normal levels of factors V and VII the reduced levels of protein C and S may lead to a thrombotic tendency (Montgomery et al 1985). However, the lower level of anti-thrombin III is commensurate with the lower levels of the vitamin K factors and this does not give rise to increased risk of thrombosis. Studies on the fibrinolytic pathway are few but suggest that in both pre-term and term infants there are reduced levels of both plasminogen and alpha 2 anti-plasmin (Beverley et al 1984c).

THE PRE-ULTRASOUND ERA

Gray et al (1968) first described the association between clotting abnor-malities and intraventricular haemorrhage. In a study of 286 low birth weight infants they found that 74 infants had a thrombotest of less than 10%, of whom 10 (14%) died of intraventricular haemorrhage. Of the remaining 212 infants only 11 (5%) died of intraventricular haemorrhage. They gave fresh frozen plasma to 26 of the 74 infants with a thrombotest of less than 10%, and only one of these infants died with an intraventricular haemor-rhage. However, nine of the remaining 48 infants who did not receive fresh frozen plasma died with an intraventricular haemorrhage. These findings were later confirmed by Thomas & Burnard (1973) who found that a concentrate of factors II, VII, IX and X reduced the incidence of intra-ventricular haemorrhage from 33% in the untreated patients to 13% in treated.

Table 4.1 Pre-ultrasound studies

Author	Conclusion
Gray 1968	Fresh frozen plasma beneficial
Thomas 1973	Factor II, VII, IX, X concentrate beneficial
Hambleton 1973	No benefit from fresh frozen plasma.
Watl 1973	No benefit from concentrate of factor II, VII, IX, X
Gupta 1976	No benefit from concentrate of factor II, VII, IX, X
Turner 1981	Coagulation defects corrected but no effect on mortality or incidence of intraventricular haemorrhage

The first controlled trial was reported in the same year by Hambleton & Appleyard (1973), who randomly assigned the infants either to treatment with fresh frozen plasma or to control groups. The authors found no beneficial effect of fresh frozen plasma on the incidence of intraventricular haemorrhage. Two other studies using a concentrate of factor II, VII, IX and X also failed to show any benefit of this product to prevent intraventricular haemorrhage (Waltl et al 1983, Gupta et al 1976). All of these studies also found difficulty in showing any consistent benefit on the underlying coagulation defect in these infants. However, Turner et al (1981) although able to demonstrate that specific coagulation defects in pre-term infants could be corrected, were unable to demonstrate any benefit in preventing intraventricular haemorrhage.

Unfortunately, all the above studies were undertaken in the pre-ultrasound era when the diagnosis of intraventricular haemorrhage was made on either clinical grounds or at post mortem. With the advent of CAT scanning and cranial ultrasonography it became apparent that many infants were developing intraventricular haemorrhages without any clinical signs whatsoever and conversely some infants who would previously have been

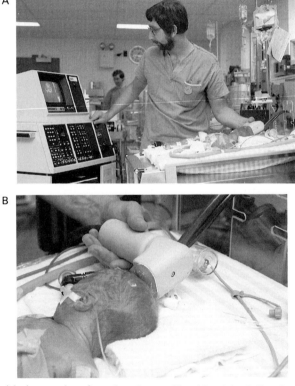

Fig. 4.1 Cranial ultrasound performed at the cot side with minimal disturbance of the infant.

thought to have had a haemorrhage on clinical grounds were, in fact, free of bleeds and had some other aetiological factor accounting for their clinical signs. Cranial ultrasound was first used in 1979 to demonstrate intraventricular haemorrhages (Pape et al 1979). Since that time it has become widely accepted as an accurate means of diagnosing intraventricular haemorrhage (Babcock and Han 1981). The procedure can be performed at the cotside through the acoustic window of the anterior fontanelle with minimal disturbance of the neonate (Fig. 4.1). The quality of the scans are such that accurate anatomical detail is revealed in both the normal (Fig. 4.2) and abnormal scan (Fig. 4.3). Many systems of grading intra-

A

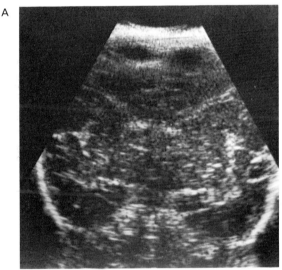

Fig. 4.2 Normal cranial ultrasound scan shown slit like lateral ventricles.

B

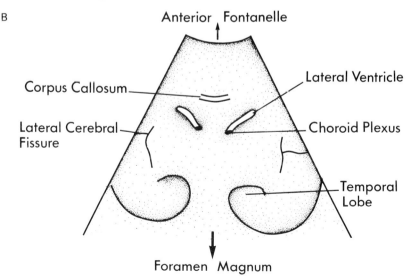

A

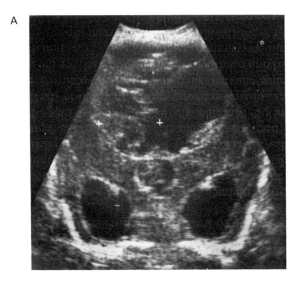

Fig. 4.3 Cranial ultrasound in an infant who has sustained a grade III intraventricular haemorrhage. There is dilatation of the body and temporal horns of the lateral ventricles and dilatation of the 3rd ventricle. Blood clot is present within the ventricular system

B

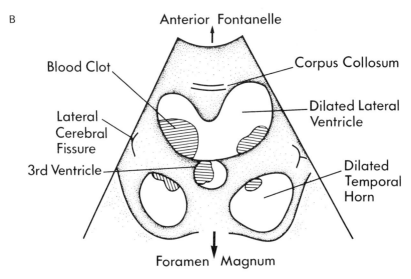

ventricular haemorrhage have been used but the one most commonly used is that of Papile et al (1978b) which was initially based on CAT scans. Their classification is as follows: Grade I – subependymal; Grade II – intraventricular without dilatation; Grade III – intraventricular with dilatation with blood; Grade IV – intracerebral or parenchymal haemorrhage.

THE ULTRASOUND ERA

In 1982 Setzer studied 58 pre-term infants using CAT scanning (Setzer et al 1982). 32 of these infants had developed periventricular or intraven-

Table 4.2 Studies using CAT scans and cranial ultrasonography

Author	Conclusion
Setzer 1982	Abnormalities of platelet function associated with intraventricular haemorrhage
Beverley 1984	Coagulation defects in cord blood associated with the development of more severe intracranial haemorrhage
McDonald 1984	Hypocoagulability in the first four hours of life associated with progression to more severe grades of intraventricular haemorrhage
Beverley 1985	Fresh frozen plasma prevents intracranial haemorrhage without any demonstrable effect on the underlying coagulation abnormality

tricular haemorrhage and in these infants they showed abnormalities of platelet function with decreased platelet counts, increased bleeding times and abnormal platelet aggregation. The authors also documented prolonged prothrombin times and activated partial thromboplastin times in these infants.

Using ultrasound, another study looked at coagulation factors in umbilical venous blood at the time of delivery and venous blood at 48 hours of age in a group of 106 pre-term infants (Beverley et al 1984d). The authors of this study showed abnormalities in coagulation at birth (Fig. 4.4) with a stepwise increase in the activated partial thromboplastin time, a stepwise

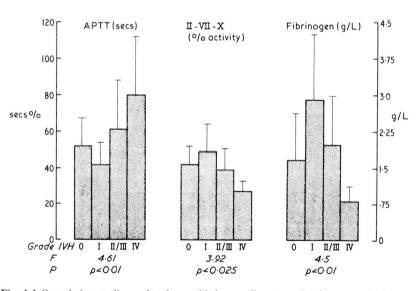

Fig. 4.4 Coagulation studies undertaken at birth according to grade of intraventricular haemorrhage. Note stepwise prolongation of APTT and stepwise decrease in % activity of factor II, VII, X and fibrinogen concentration according to the severity of haemorrhage. (Results expressed as mean + 1 S.D. After Beverley et al 1984d.)

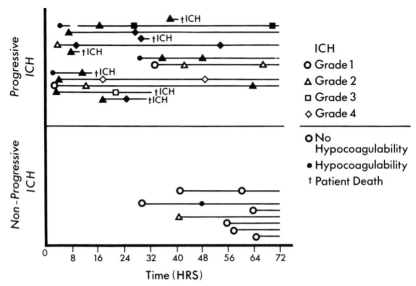

Fig. 4.5 Progressive extension of intracranial haemorrhage (ICH) relative to the presence of hypocoagulability. (Reproduced by permission of *Paediatrics* from McDonald et al 1984.)

fall in the per cent activity of factors II, VII and X and a stepwise fall in the fibrinogen concentration according to the severity of haemorrhage. It is also interesting to note that the coagulation status of the infants sustaining grade one haemorrhages was better than those developing no haemorrhage, which suggests that the more efficient clotting system in those with grade one haemorrhage was able to limit any minor capillary leak. By 48 h of age these abnormalities were reported as persisting; in addition there were further abnormalities of haemostasis in those infants sustaining the more severe haemorrhages with a fall in platelet count and a rise in the mean platelet volume. The abnormalities of coagulation described at birth and age 48 h could not be accounted for by prematurity alone as the values quoted were outside the normal ranges for that laboratory.

Later that year, McDonald et al (1984) were able to substantiate the above study showing that many infants who developed intraventricular haemorrhage had hypocoagulable blood with lower values for fibrinogen, platelet count, antithrombin III and factor VIII and higher values for fibrin monomer and longer Laidlaw whole blood clotting times. They were also able to show that hypocoagulability during the first four hours of life was associated with progression to more severe grades of intraventricular haemorrhage (Fig. 4.5).

PREVENTION OF INTRAVENTRICULAR HAEMORRHAGE

Recent follow up studies have determined the long term neurological sequelae of intraventricular haemorrhage (Shankaran et al 1982). The largest study by Papile et al (1983) showed that whilst only 15% of pre-term infants having no or only grade I or II haemorrhages had major or multiple handicaps, 50% of those infants sustaining grade III and 86% of those with grade IV haemorrhages had major or multiple handicaps. It is with these long term sequelae in mind that various therapeutic maneouvres have been tried to prevent intraventricular haemorrhage. As discussed at the start of this chapter, the most important of these have been the maintenance of the blood gases and arterial blood pressure, thereby preventing rapid changes in cerebral blood flow.

Various drugs have been used to try and prevent intraventricular haemorrhage. Ethamsylate (Morgan et al 1981) which increases platelet adhesion and acts on local thromboplastin release and reinforces the capillary basement membrane has been found to be of particular benefit. In a study of 70 pre-term infants, 18 of 35 control patients compared with 9 of 35 treated patients developed intraventricular haemorrhage. It has been reported that phenobarbitone has a protective effect (Donn et al 1981) but this work has not been supported by other authors (Kuban et al 1986). Vitamin E (20 mg/kg i.m. at birth, 24 h and 48 h), a potent antioxidant and membrane stabiliser, has been shown to have a beneficial effect in preventing intraventricular haemorrhage. In the original report Chiswick et al (1983) showed that supplementation with vitamin E had a marked effect (Fig. 4.6), and more recently they reported the result of a randomized study on 226 newborn babies in which the incidence of intraventricular haemorrhage was reduced from 40% to 9.1% in treated patients (Chiswick et al 1986).

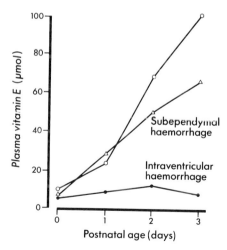

Fig. 4.6 Median plasma vitamin E concentrations at different postnatal ages in babies < 32 weeks gestation without any haemorrhages (O), with subependymal haemorrhage only (▲) and with intraventricular haemorrhage (●). (Reproduced with kind permission from Chiswick et al 1983.)

The mechanism of action of vitamin E in preventing intraventricular haemorrhage is poorly understood. One function of vitamin E is to protect the cell membranes against lipid peroxidation. Chiswick et al (1983) proposed in their original paper that oxidative damage to capillary endothelial membranes of the subependymal layer contributed to the occurrence of intraventricular haemorrhage and vitamin E protected against this oxidative damage.

In support of this hypothesis they cite three examples. Firstly, intraventricular haemorrhage is relatively uncommon in stillborn babies where it is known that the foetal PaO_2 is normally only 3.3 KPa. Secondly vitamin E deficient chickens develop a condition called nutritional encephalomalacia which is associated with spontaneous haemorrhage into the cerebellum and elsewhere in the central nervous system, and finally in hamsters there is a vitamin E responsive condition known as spontaneous haemorrhagic disease of the central nervous system in which the initial haemorrhagic lesions do involve the subependymal vasculature and progress to intraventricular haemorrhage. Despite the excellent results reported, it must be remembered that vitamin E is not without its side effects; vitamin E has been associated with increased fibrinolysis and platelet aggregation and the oral preparation has been associated with outbreaks of necrotizing enterocolitis. Also the parenteral preparation had to be withdrawn in 1984 in the USA because of major hepatic, renal and haemopoietic toxicity and deaths in 38 infants receiving the drug (Aranda et al 1986).

The effect of fresh frozen plasma has recently been recorded (Beverley et al 1985). In this study 73 infants less than 1500 g and/or less than 32 weeks gestation were studied. The patients were randomly assigned to receive treatment with fresh frozen plasma (10 ml/kg on admission and 10 ml/kg at 24 h of age) or to control groups. The two study populations were well-matched for factors that had previously been noted to be associated with the development of intraventricular haemorrhage and, in particular, there was no difference in the coagulation parameters measured at the time of entry into the trial. The results showed a reduction in incidence of intraventricular haemorrhage from 41% in the control infants to 14% in those receiving fresh frozen plasma. However, there was no beneficial effect in terms of coagulation parameters for, when the clotting studies were repeated at 48 h of age, there was no difference between the control and treated groups. The authors discuss whether the beneficial effect of fresh frozen plasma that they described was mediated through the coagulation cascade or through some other mechanism such as stabilization of the systemic arterial blood pressure.

OTHER TYPES OF INTRACRANIAL HAEMORRHAGE

Although intraventricular haemorrhage is the predominant type of intracranial haemorrhage, other types of intracranial bleeds do occur.

Subdural haemorrhage

Subdural haemorrhage is the least common variety of intracranial haemorrhage and is predominantly traumatic in origin (Craig 1939). Haemorrhages usually occur when delivery of a relatively large head occurs through a small birth canal or when there is rapid deformation of the skull during a precipitant delivery. The major sites of bleeding are from the straight sinus, vein of Galen and lateral sinus when the tentorium is lacerated; the occipital sinus when there is occipital diastasis; and the inferior sagittal sinus when there is rupture of the falx. The diagnosis is dependant on the clinical history with signs referable to the brain stem suggesting a posterior fossa haemorrhage, whilst focal signs such as a hemiparesis would suggest a supratentorial collection of blood. The diagnosis can be assisted by subdural taps. Diagnostic imaging with CAT scans confirm the diagnosis. Unfortunately, the prognosis for these infants with lacerations of the falx and tentorium is nearly always uniformly fatal though the outlook for those infants with convexity haematomas is more favourable.

Cerebellar haemorrhages

These have been described as being associated with birth trauma (Pape and Wigglesworth 1979) and bleeding diathesis (Chessells and Wigglesworth 1976) but in the majority of cases many of the same factors as associated with intraventricular haemorrhage are present. The vascular integrity within the cerebellum is poor (Pape and Wigglesworth 1979) and germinal matrix is present around the fourth ventricle so that in the face of poor autoregulation haemorrhage is likely to occur. One other association that has been particularly noted with the cerebellar haemorrhage is that of face mask ventilation. Pape et al (1976) noted that with this form of artificial ventilation the strapping that held the mask in place caused deformation of the occipital bone with subsequent cerebellar haemorrhage.

Subarachnoid haemorrhage

This is a common cause of finding blood in the cerebro-spinal fluid at the time of lumbar puncture. In one series 29% of children with blood in the cerebro-spinal fluid had a primary subarachnoid haemorrhage and 63% had intraventricular haemorrhages (Volpe 1981). The aetiology of subarachnoid haemorrhage in neonates is poorly understood but is thought to be of traumatic origin in term infants and due to 'hypoxic' insults in the pre-term baby. Usually the signs of haemorrhage are minimal in the majority of infants but occasionally the child may present with apneoic spells or convulsions. Fortunately, the prognosis is excellent and is determined by the nature of the insult that caused the haemorrhage rather than the haemorrhage itself.

Bleeding disorders presenting as intracranial haemorrhage

It is rare for primary bleeding disorders to present with intracranial haemorrhage alone; there are usually signs of bleeding at sites other than the central nervous system. Patients with severe haemophillia have presented with any of the types of intracranial haemorrhage discussed. Vitamin K deficiency, particularly in the breast fed baby, may present with a variety of intracranial haemorrhages depending on the perinatal complications that the infant may have experienced. Isoimmune thrombocytopenia may lead to subrachnoid haemorrhage in 15–20% of cases (Pearson et al 1964) but fortunately intracerebral haemorrhage is much less common. Disseminated intravascular coagulation is not an uncommon occurrence in the sick pre-term infant (Oski and Naiman 1982) and usually presents with oozing from venepuncture sites. However, bleeding can occur at any location and intracranial haemorrhage may be a problem. The treatment for these specific coagulation disorders is directed at correcting the underlying abnormality with the use of the appropriate blood transfusion product.

CONCLUSIONS

Intraventricular haemorrhage is the most common type of neonatal intracranial haemorrhage. Its aetiology is multifactorial but it would seem apparent from the data published, in both the pre-ultrasound and ultrasound era, that there is a strong association between coagulation abnormalities and the occurrence of intraventricular haemorrhage. Recent studies have shown that therapeutic interventions with ethamsylate and vitamin E can decrease the incidence of bleeds and hopefully, therefore, the neurological sequelae. Fresh frozen plasma seems to have a beneficial effect in preventing intraventricular haemorrhage though a larger study is needed to determine its mode of action and also to ascertain whether other agents such as cryoprecipitate or albumin may have a more beneficial effect. A study similar to that orginally described by Turner et al (1981), but repeated using ultrasound, may be the way forward to answering this question. As yet there is no completely safe therapy that is available to prevent intraventricular haemorrhage. Vitamin E, though extremely efficacious, is not without its toxic side effects and the transfusion of blood products is associated with the known hazards of hepatitis and AIDS. At the present time therapeutic intervention will have to be assessed by the risk versus the potential benefits to the patients. Long term follow up studies will determine whether any of the interventions described ultimately effects the neurological outcome of these pre-term infants.

Acknowledgements

I would like to thank the Department of Medical Illustration at St James's University Hospital for help in preparing the illustrations and Mrs Christine Silburn who typed the manuscript.

REFERENCES

Allan W C, Volpe J J 1986 Periventricular-intraventricular haemorrhage. Pediatric Clinics of North America 33: 47–63

Aranda J V, Chemtob S, Laudignon N, Sasyniuk B 1986 Furosemide and vitamin E, two problem drugs in neonatology. Pediatric Clinics of North America 33: 583–602

Babcock D S , Han B K 1981 The accuracy of high resolution real time ultrasonography of the head in infancy. Radiology 139: 665–676

Beverley D W, Chance G W, Coates C F 1984a Intraventricular haemorrhage – timing of occurrence and relationship to perinatal events. British Journal of Obstetrics and Gynaecolgy 91: 1007–1013

Beverley D W, Chance G W 1984b Cord blood gases, birth asphyxia and intraventricular haemorrhage. Archives of Diseases in Childhood 59: 884–887

Beverley D W, Inwood M J, Chance G W, Schaus M, O'Keefe B 1984c Normal haemostasis parameters: a study in a well defined inborn population of pre-term infants. Early Human Development 9: 249–257

Beverley D W, Chance G W, Inwood M J, Schaus M, O'Keefe B 1984d Intraventricular haemorrhage and haemostasis defects. Archives of Diseases in Childhood 59: 444–448

Beverley D W, Pitts-Tucker T J, Congdon P J, Arthur R J, Tate G 1985 Prevention of intraventricular haemorrhage by fresh frozen plasma. Archives of Diseases in Childhood 60: 710–713

Buchanan G R 1986 Coagulation disorders in the neonate. Pediatric Clinics of North America 33: 203–220

Clarke C E, Clyman R I, Roth R S et al 1981 Risk factor analysis of intraventricular haemorrhage in low birth weight infants. Journal of Pediatrics 99: 625–628

Cooke R W I 1981 Factors associated with periventricular haemorrhage in very low birth weight infants. Archives of Diseases in Childhood 56: 425–431

Chessells J M, Wigglesworth J S 1970 Secondary haemorrhagic disease of the newborn. Archives of Diseases in Childhood 45: 539–543

Chiswick M L, Johnson M, Woodhall C et al 1983 Protective effect of vitamin E against intraventricular haemorrhage in premature babies. British Medical Journal 287: 81–84

Chiswick M L, Sinha S, Davies J, Sims D G 1986 Vitamin E protects against periventricular haemorrhage in per-term babies. Presented at the Annual Meeting of the British Paediatric Association, York, 1986

Craig W S 1939 Intracranial haemorrhage in the newborn. Archive of Diseases in Childhood 13: 89–94

Donat J F, Okazaki H, Kleinberg F, Reagan T J 1978 Intraventricular haemorrhages in full term and premature infants. Mayo Clinic Proceedings 53: 437–442

Donn S M, Roloff D W, Goldstein G W 1981 Prevention of intraventricular haemorrhage in pre-term infants by phenobarbitone. Lancet II: 215–217

Fedrick J, Butler N R 1970 Certain causes of neonatal death, II Intraventricular haemorrhage. Biology of the Neonate 15: 257–290

Fujimura M, Salisbury D M, Robinson R O et al 1979 Clinical events relating to intraventricular haemorrhage in the newborn. Archives of Diseases in Childhood 54: 409–414

Giles F H, Price R A, Kevy S V et al 1971 Fibrinolytic activity in the ganlionic eminence of the premature human brain. Biology of the Neonate 18: 426–432

Gray O P, Ackerman A, Fraser J A 1968 Intracranial haemorrhage and clotting defects in low birth weight babies. Lancet I: 545–548

Grunewald P 1957 Subependymal cerebral haemorrhage in premature infants, and its relation to various injurious influences at birth. American Journal of Obstetrics and Gynaecology 61: 1285–1292

Gupta J M, Starr H, Fincher P, Lam-Po-Tang P R L C 1976 Intraventricular haemorrhage in the newborn. Medical Journal of Australia 2: 338–340

Hambleton G, Appleyard W J 1973 Controlled trial of fresh frozen plasma in asphyxiated low birth weight infants. Archives of Diseases in Childhood 48: 31–35

Hambleton G, Wigglesworth J S 1976 Origin of intraventricular haemorrhage in the pre-term infant. Archives of Diseases in Childhood 51: 651–659

Hill A, Perlman J M, Volpe J J 1982 Relationship of pneumothorax to the occurrence of intraventricular haemorrhage in the premature newborn. Pediatrics 69: 144–149

Kenny J D, Garcia Prats J A, Hilliard J L et al 1978 Hypercarbia at birth: a possible role in the pathogenesis of intraventricular haemorrhage. Pediatrics 62: 465–467

Kuban K C K, Leviton A, Krishnamoorthy K S et al 1986 Neonatal intracranial haemorrhage and Phenobarbital. Pediatrics 77: 443–450

Levine M I, Fawer C L, Lamong R F 1982 Risk factors in the development of intraventricular haemorrhage in the pre-term infant. Archives of Diseases in Childhood 57: 410–417

Lipscomb A P , Reynolds E O R, Blackwell R J et al 1981 Pneumothorax and cerebral haemorrhage in pre-term infants. Lancet 1: 414–416

Lou H C, Lassen W A, Friis-Hansen B 1979a Impaired autoregulation of cerebral blood flow in the distressed newborn infant. Journal of Pediatrics 94: 118–121

Lou H C, Lassen W A, Tweed W A, 1979b Pressure positive cerebral blood flow and breakdown of blood brain barrier in experimental fetal asphyxia. Acta Pediatrica Scandinavica 68: 57–63

McDonald M M, Johnson M L, Rumack C M et al 1984 Role of coagulopathy in newborn intracranial haemorrhage. Pediatrics 74: 26–31

Montgomery R R, Marlar R A, Gill J C 1985 Newborn haemostasis. Clinical Studies in Haemotology 14: 443–460

Morgan M E I, Benson J W T, Cooke R W I 1981 Ethamsylate reduces in the incidence of perventricular haemorrhage in very low birth weight babeis. Lancet II: 830–831

Oski F A, Naiman J L 1981 Haematological problems in the newborn. 3rd Ed. W B Saunders, Philadelphia

Pape K E, Armstrong D L, Fitzharding P M 1976 Central nervous system pathology associated with mask ventilation in the very low birthweight infant: a new etiology for intracerebellar haemorrhages. Pediatrics 58: 473–483

Pape K E, Wigglesworth J S 1979a Haemorrhage, ischaemia and the perinatal brain. Lippincott, Philadelphia

Pape K E, Cusick G, Houang M T W et al 1979b Ultrasound detection of brain damage in pre-term infants. Lancet I: 1261–1263

Papile L, Burstein J, Burstein R, 1978a Relationship of intravenous sodium bicarbonate infusions and cerebral intraventricular haemorrhage. Journal of Pediatrics 93: 834–839

Papile L, Burstein J, Burstein R, Koffler H 1978b Incidence and evolution of subependymal haemorrhage: a study of infants with birth weight less than 1 500 mgs. Journal of Pediatrics 92: 529–534

Papile L A, Munsich-Bruno G, Shaefer A 1983 Relationship of cerebral intraventricular haemorrhage and early childhood neurological handicaps. Journal of Pediatrics 103: 273–277

Pearson H A, Shulman N R, Marder V J, Cone T E 1964 Isoimmune neonatal thrombocytopenic purpura. Blood 23: 154–159

Perlman J M, McMenamin J B, Volpe J J, 1983 Fluctuating cerebral blood flow velocity in respiratory distress syndrome: relation to the development of intracranial haemorrhage. New England Journal of Medicine 309: 204–209

Setzer E S, Webb I B, Wassenaar J W et al 1982 Platelet dysfunction and coagulopathy in intraventricular haemorrhage in the premature infant. Journal of Pediatrics 100: 599–605

Shankaran S, Slovis T L, Bedard M P, Poland R L 1982 Sonographic classification of intracranial haemorrhage. A prognostic indicator of mortality, morbidity and short term neurological outcome. Journal of Pediatrics 100: 469–475

Stuart M J 1979 Platelet function in the nconate. American Journal of Pediatric Haematology and Oncology 1: 227–234

Tarby T J, Volpe J J 1982 Intraventricular haemorrhage in the premature infant. Pediatric Clinics of North America 29: 1077–1104

Thomas D B, Burnard E D 1973 Prevention of intraventricular haemorrhage in babies receiving artificial ventilation. Medical Journal of Australia I: 933–936

Turner T, Prowse C V, Prescott R J, Cash J D 1981 A clinical trial of the early detection and connection of haemostatic defects in selected high risk neonates. British Journal of Haematology 47: 65–75

Volpe J J 1981a Neonatal intraventricular haemorrhage. New England Journal of Medicine 304: 886–91

Volpe J J 1981b Neurology of the newborn. Saunders, Philadelphia

Waltl H, Kurtz R̄, Mitterstieler G et al 1973 Intracranial haemorrhage in low birth weight infants and prophylactic administration of coagulation-factor concentrate. Lancet I: 1284–1286

Yakovlev P I, Rosales R K 1970 Distribution of the terminal haemorrhages in the brain wall in stillborn premature and non viable neonates. In: Physical trauma as an etiologic agent in nental retardation. US Government Printing Office, Washington

Ylppö A 1919 Beitrage zur Physiologie, Pathologie, und sozialen Hygiene dea Kindersalters. Pathologisch-anatomische Sludien bei Fruhgeburten. Springer. Berlin

Machine options for apheresis

INTRODUCTION

Since the early animal experimental work in 1914 of John Abel (Abel et al 1914) at John's Hopkins Medical School in Baltimore, plasmapheresis has received much attention.

Although the manual technique of plasmapheresis is still widely practised for the collection of donor plasma its use for therapeutic plasmapheresis is not widely used, since time and volume are major restrictive factors.

The development of machines for haemapheresis originates from the work of Edwin Cohn at Harvard University, Boston. He introduced, in the 1940s, an adapted model E-19 De Laval cream separator for the separation of large quantities of plasma and the concept of mechanical blood separation was born. An important step forward was the development of the ADL Cohn Blood Fractionator by the Cohn group under the direction of Allan Latham Jr, in close cooperation with Arthur D Little, Cambridge, Massachusetts. Further engineering developments led to the construction of a simplified reusable bowl, mounted in an IEC PR-2 centrifuge for the separation of plasma from whole blood (Tullis et al 1956). Tullis (Tullis et al 1971) further developed the concept into the prototype of the present bowl and compact drive equipment, the Haemonetics discontinuous flow centrifugation model 10, which was introduced in the mid 1960s.

Almost simultaneously a continuous flow centrifugation principle was developed by Eisel and Freireich at the Cancer Institute, Houston, Texas in close co-operation with George Judson, project engineer with International Business Machines Inc. (Freireich et al 1965). This principle was designed primarily for the collection of granulocytes and resulted in the construction of the NCI-IBM continuous flow centrifugation blood cell separator, a machine which was made available for field trials in 1966.

With the same purpose in mind Djerassi et al (1970) developed the principle of continuous blood flow through nylon fibre filters for apheresis of leucocytes from donors. In this ingenious noncentrifugal system the white cells are first entrapped by the nylon fibres and subsequently eluted for transfusion. Although this technique yields a significant number of granulocytes, adverse effects of the nylon fibres on cell morphology and function have been observed and the technique has now been abandoned.

Following the developments in haemodialysis, plasma filtration through porous membranes was devised in the late 1970s (Solomon et al 1978) as a means for separating plasma from blood cells and hollow fibres have been introduced widely in continuous flow systems, primarily for therapeutic plasma exchange. In the early 1980's both centrifugation and filtration principles were moulded into a revolutionary new and admirably elegant design, enabling the harvesting of plasma as well as platelets from donors in a discontinuous flow system.

APHERESIS POSSIBILITIES

The term apheresis was first introduced by Abel using the Greek word 'αφαιρεσις', meaning withdraw. The word was used in conjunction with the component to be withdrawn: plasmapheresis.

In relation to blood, apheresis can be applied to the removal or withdrawal of specific components like plasma, platelets, granulocytes or stem cells from donors. Alternatively, the removal of unwanted substances, considered to be pathogenic in certain diseases, can be apheresed from the patient's circulating blood.

Donor haemapheresis

For the harvesting of large quantities of a specific blood component from one individual donor, haemapheresis is now widely accepted and applied within blood banks. The development of the concept originates from the second world war when the need for plasma to combat haemorrhagic shock urged the exploration of human plasmapheresis. Although the development of machine apheresis emerged from the early efforts to collect and process large quantities of plasma, the option for mechanical plasmapheresis from donors was not explored until the 1980's.

The machines constructed were primarily used for the harvesting of granulocytes and platelets for supportive haemotherapy in leukaemia and oncology patients.

Plasma collection by mechanical apheresis can be done by centrifugation, filtration or combined centrifugation and filtration. Plasma can be collected for routine fractionation into the full range of purified protein components or for the harvesting of specific immune plasmas, such as anti-D, anti-tetanus or anti-CMV.

Cell collection by mechanical apheresis follows exclusively the centrifugation principle. The major objective is the harvesting of sufficient amounts of cells from a single donor to allow adequate transfusion therapy. This reduces the risk of transmitting diseases and the exposure to foreign anti-gens, therefore optimising the supportive haemotherapy. The potential for specific cell collections include platelets, granulocytes, neocytes and pluri-potent stem cells.

In donor haemapheresis the use of machines has provided the option to increase safety, purity, potency and efficacy of harvested components. However, the introduction of extracorporeal circuits in donor procedures also has given potential problems and hazards (Huestis et al 1981). Biocom-patibility of software and the physico-mechanical processing of the blood is of paramount importance for preserving optimal plasma protein and cell function. Activation of enzyme and complement systems is an almost unavoidable consequence. In the desire to harvest more and higher quality of cells or plasma proteins, drugs have been introduced to stimulate physio-logic mechanisms in the donor. Here the developments have not always been tested against the ethical principles of a voluntary blood donation.

Therapeutic haemapheresis

Haemapheresis has now been accepted as a mode to remove unwanted patho-logic components from the blood of a patient in order to support the treat-ment of a specific disease. Another indication for therapeutic haemapheresis is the administration of an essential plasma substance in the context of restrictions with regard to volume replacement. Therapeutic haemapheresis has been reported in a wide variety of clinical specialities. These include haematology and oncology, immunology, nephrology, rheumatology, neurology and dermatology. Therapeutic haemapheresis is currently prac-tised to remove or reduce the number of peripheral white cells in patients with leukaemia, platelets in patients with thrombocythaemia and red cells in patients with sickle cell crisis.

Plasma exchange is the most widely practised type of therapeutic haemapheresis. Therapeutic plasma exchange had a slow start after the early machines became available in the mid 1960's. However, in the 1970's the use of therapeutic plasma exchange exploded and became an almost uncon-trollable growth area. The list of pathologic conditions thought to be eligible for plasma exchange extended almost daily. However, the funda-mental criteria for assessing possible benefits from therapeutic haemapher-esis are the evidence that the patient's disease or its symptomatology may be due to or aggravated by an abnormal plasma constituent or a deficiency of a normal plasma constituent, or the presence of pathologic blood cells both in type and number.

The possible mechanisms by which therapeutic plasma exchange could be of benefit to patients are the removal of autoantibodies, alloantibodies, circulating antigens or immunecomplexes, monoclonal proteins or protein bound toxins. In some diseases the replacement of a specific but undefined factor is believed to be the mechanism, such as in thrombotic thrombocytopenic purpura. In only a very limited number of diseases has the postulated mechanism been established scientifically.

The removal of unwanted cells, as for instance in leukocytaemia's and sickle cell crisis, follows the principle of cell collection in donor cytapheresis. To separate the unwanted cells from the blood, centrifugation is applied in a continuous or discontinuous flow system.

Therapeutic plasma exchange has been done by centrifugation or filtration methods. In principle the plasma is exchanged by a replacement fluid. The efficacy of this rather crude approach depends on a variety of factors:

a. levels of the unwanted substance in the intravascular compartment
b. exchange rate of the unwanted substance between intravascular and extravascular compartment and vice versa
c. synthesis rate of the unwanted substance
d. catabolism of the unwanted substance.

The clinical benefit may require a lower plasma constituent level than that which can be achieved by plasma exchange. If we assume that the plasma constituent to be eliminated is the principle pathogenic factor and that the value of synthesis, catabolism and compartmental exchange are all equal to zero, then the disappearance curve of plasma constituents during a therapeutic exchange can be calculated by linear regression of the Ln transformed values plotted against the number of plasma volumes removed (Derksen 1983). This hypothetical ideal physical model curve will then be a straight line. Further analysis of the model, on the basis of plasma volume calculation of the patient, has shown that a 1–1.5 plasma volume exchange offers optimal efficacy. Exchange volumes beyond 1.5 plasma volume do not contribute beneficially in terms of the effort and costs required to achieve a larger volume, due to the diluting effect of the replacement fluid.

Once the plasma is removed by centrifugation or filtration, a cascade principle for a specific elimination of factors can be applied (Pineda & Taswell 1981). Studies are now in progress, using a series of filters of different pore sizes, for the elimination of specific proteins like macromolecules or using interconnected affinity columns which specifically adsorb metabolites, immune complexes, circulating antibodies or other unwanted organic substances. The interconnection of a cold insoluble globulin precipitating chamber potentially allows removal of cryoglobulins. For the development of all these principles, a more precise understanding of the pathophysiology of the relevant diseases is still needed. Without this the options for new machine apheresis developments for therapeutic haemapheresis cannot be easily explored and subsequently developed. Nonetheless existing mechanical apheresis technology does provide a potentially useful tool to support the treatment of a variety of patients, predominantly with autoimmune diseases. In a limited amount of time large quantities of plasma constituents considered to be of relevance for the course of the disease, can be removed and replaced by a fluid of choice.

The inevitable extracorporeal circuit and the need for replacing fluids, render the technique potentially hazardous. The risk factors in general can be defined as follows:

a. machine and software
b. personnel and procedure
c. indication and patient condition.

Therapeutic haemapheresis has been developed in many centres physically distant from the clinical environs. This can be a cause for concern when seriously ill patients require apheresis procedures. Whatever the location for therapeutic haemapheresis, the personnel must be committed to optimal patient care and continuous education, training and familiarity with apheresis machines. Techniques and recognition of potential problems are vitally important.

PRINCIPLES OF MECHANICAL HAEMAPHERESIS

Since the introduction of mechnical blood separators, two main principles for haemapheresis have been developed (Smit Sibinga 1986).

1. The centrifugation principle – the technique follows either a continuous or discontinuous flow principle.
2. The filtration principle – the technique is an analogue of haemodialysis and usually incorporates a continuous flow mode.

Both principles are based on the processing of blood in an extracorporeal circuit. The blood is passed vein-to-vein through the extracorporeal circuit and subjected to an artificial manipulative process: more or less modified blood is then returned. The biotechnical problems of extracorporeal circuit technology relate to the biocompatibility of the necessary constituents, the effect of blood pumps and flow rates, the control of the extracorporeal volume and the inevitable anticoagulation. The requirements for mechanical haemapheresis devices are based on donor or patient safety, maintenance of sterility, disposable integral blood pathway of optimal biocompatibility, ease of operation and maintenance, versatility and portability, reliability and an acceptable cost-benefit ratio.

Centrifugation principle

Blood can be processed for cell or plasma separation by centrifugation using a discontinuous or intermittent flow technique, or a continuous flow technique. The latter technique requires a two vein access, whereas the former needs only one arm, as both collection and return are carried out through the same needle. Both techniques are based on the collection and simultaneous separation of blood in a rotating chamber, requiring a compact drive mechanism. The separation takes place through differences in specific gravity of the blood constituents, harvesting the separated component at appropriate time intervals and by channelling a particular layer into a collection bag. The remaining processed blood is then returned. Anti-coagulation is usually achieved by a citrate medium, ACD being used in most procedures at a variety of anticoagulant-to-blood ratios.

Discontinuous flow centrifugation (DFC)

The original concept of discontinuous flow centrifugation for haemapheresis was developed by Latham and Kingsley (1975). The separation chamber is a rotating bowl, mounted on a centrifuge plateau. The neck of the bowl is fixed and connected to the bowl by a rotating seal. The blood flows into the bowl from the top, is channelled down to the bottom and then centri-fuged outwards and upwards into the separation chamber of the rotating bowl. The harvesting is done from the top outwards into a connection bag. The rotating seal is the weakest point of this otherwise mechanically simple, versatile and disposable system. The two major problems are the sterility and the control of heat generation during the centrifugation process. The equipment, as developed and worldwide marketed by Haemonetics, allows collection of platelets and granulocytes as well as plasma. The original model 10 has been succeeded by the model 30, which is still in regular service in many haemapheresis units all over the world. The third gener-ation, evolved out of the desire to simplify the somewhat unpractical shape of the main frame, is the model 30S. It is a more compact and shorter version, still functioning on a manual operating basis.

Automation of the collection, separation, harvesting and return stages of the haemapheresis process has been achieved in the V50 model. This fourth generation machine is programmable and detects the principle separation layers, plasma, buffy coat and red cells, by optical detectors. The machine can be operated fully automatic but has the option for manual control. Further developments have concentrated on the elimination of contami-nating white cells and red cells from platelets. The principle of this devel-opment is based on a hydrodynamic step in the buffy coat collection. When the buffy coat reaches the shoulder of the bowl it is optically detected, the drawing of blood from the donor is then stopped, while the rotating speed of the centrifuge remains constant. A surge pump is activated, reinjecting at high speed autologous plasma into the spinning bowl. This results in resolution of the platelets from the white cells and red cells in the buffy coat (elutriative surge effect). The valve to the collection bag is then auto-matically opened to harvest the platelets, which have been boosted away from the remaining buffy coat fraction, providing a significantly purer platelet concentrate (Schoendorfer et al 1983). Since the introduction of the surge principle for plateletapheresis, much research has been done to further elucidate the hydrodynamic process. The success of the technique very much depends on donor variables such as haematocrit, platelet count and clarity of the plasma, as well as on machine variables (Elias et al 1985). The latter specifically depends on the way plasma reinjection speed is built up, the maximum surge speed, the optical detection of the elutriated purified platelet rich plasma and the braking of the surge process determining the endpoint of the harvesting procedure (Van Ede 1985).

Platelet elutriation is currently in its third generation development, allowing a fully automated microprocessor controlled harvesting of a red cell depleted platelet concentrate, contaminated with an acceptable minimum number of white cells, almost exclusively lymphocytes.

The shape of the processing chamber in the bowl has also been adapted in order to influence the hydrodynamic flow patterns of the blood constituent layers in the spinning bowl and to counteract the comparatively large extracorporeal volume. Originally, there were large (375 ml) and small (225 ml) bowls. To reduce the extracorporeal volume, a 110 ml pediatric bowl has been developed. To optimize the processing chamber and reduce the volume, a grenade bowl of different geometry has also been designed.

The machine options in the rotating bowl DFC principle are limited to Haemonetics and Dideco. Haemonetics markets, for cytapheresis and therapeutic haemapheresis purposes, the 30S and V50 series of automated microprocessor controlled machines. A modification, designed specifically for donor plasmapheresis, is the plasma collection system or PCS. By varying the centrifugation speed either a platelet rich plasma at low speed or a platelet poor plasma at higher speed can be harvested. The Haemonetics PCS machine is fully automated and requires very little operator assistance. The technique is based on a single needle principle allowing the collection of 500 ml plasma in 28–40 min (needle in to needle out).

Dideco markets the BT790, a semiautomated machine which is very similar in principle to the Haemonetics model 30 equipment. There are differences in design of both hardware and software, but in essence the machine is a replica of the Haemonetics disposable bowl and compact motordrive system. The Dideco equipment is used for cytapheresis and therapeutic haemapheresis.

For donor plasmapheresis two other DFC principles have been recently developed.
1. the belt or toroid shaped separation chamber
2. the cylinder shaped spinning membrane filtration system.

MSE have developed the SPC 600 automated donor plasmapheresis machine. The SPC 600 software set has a belt shaped or 'toroidal' separation chamber, very similar to the belt shaped original IBM 2997 single channel system. The method enables good separation of plasma to be achieved without exposing blood to high sheer rates. The SPC donor set has no rotating seals and the machine is microprocessor controlled, with the option to override the automatic control sequence to pause, complete or to stop the procedure.

HemaScience developed the Autopheresis-C device, which is a fully automated machine for donor plasmapheresis. The principle is based on an extremely ingenious combination of centrifugation and filtration. The separation chamber is cylinder shaped, with a membrane mounted in a rotating inner cylinder and a fixed outer wall. The rotation is driven by a magnet system, avoiding an 'open' rotating seal. Blood flows from the top into the vertically positioned separation chamber. The red cells are centrifugally driven away from the spinning membrane and the plasma then passes easily through the membrane into the inner cylinder and is collected downwards into a collection bag. The red cells leave the separation chamber at the bottom and are temporarily stored in a reinfusion chamber. The constant rotation of the membrane increases the filtration efficacy since the turbulance tends to prevent membrane clogging and cell build up. The effective surface area is only 0.005 m² with a processing volume of 7 ml. The machine is microprocessor operated and extremely user friendly, as can be experienced from the low alarm rate during processing. The software is designed for the collection of plasma in a single needle discontinuous flow system. The collection of 500 ml plasma takes 25–35 min (needle in to needle out).

Continuous flow centrifugation (CFC)

The continuous flow centrifugation principle as designed by Mr Robert Eisel and Dr Emil J. Freireich in close co-operation with International Business Machines Inc., was primarily developed for granulocyte harvesting (Freireich et al 1965). The first operational machine was the NCI-IBM 2990 blood cell separator. This model and the Aminco Celltrifuge I apparatus operate through intricate reusable bowls, which must be disassembled for cleaning and sterilizing in between use. They have the major disadvantage of being extremely difficult to clean effectively and therefore carry the potential risk for transmitting viral diseases. Some of these older machines are still in use. The Aminco Celltrifuge I was further improved by Fenwal and the Celltrifuge II is an excellent machine with a disposable blood processing software. However, IBM have totally redesigned their original continuous flow centrifugation concept. The centrifuge-mounted fixed separation chamber, where the blood flows during separation parallel to the axis of rotation, has been replaced by a rotating belt or hoop-like disposable software channel with a component separation and collection chamber (Hester et al 1979). This single stage separation channel differs in two important ways from the so far developed CFC and DFC systems. The blood flow during separation is circumferential instead of axial. Secondly, the interface position within the channel is stabilized by the special design of the collection chamber, so that only minimal operator attention is required. The operator can observe the separation and collection chamber while rotating by means of a strobe light. This IBM 2997 single channel CFC system is extremely suitable for therapeutic plasma exchange. For granulocyte and platelet collection this device has the disadvantage of requiring close attention and constant adjustments by the operator.

A variation on this concept has been developed by Dideco. The BT 798 Viva follows the same principle, although there are marked differences in the design of the instrument and the disposable separator set. This machine is specifically designed for therapeutic plasma exchange. Whole blood flows into the belt-shaped separation chamber that ends in a wedge-shaped collection chamber which is perpendicularly positioned on the belt. Red cells are collected through the outer part of the wedge-shaped collection chamber where the plasma is harvested through an outlet at the inner corner of the collection chamber. The centrifuge housing has a built-in blood warming system to prevent cryoproteins from precipitation during the separation process. Attached to the main frame is an automatic fluid balance system assuring a perfect balance between collected plasma and reinfused replacement fluids.

Another variation has been developed by the Japanese Green Cross Corporation. This continuous plasmapheresis centrifuge machine operates entirely automatically. The software design is a completely closed system. The operation can be monitored by a special stroboscope, which enables observation of the spinning separator. Although initially designed for plasma separation at a capacity of 200 ml/h, the device can also be used for leucocyte and platelet collections.

The circumferential flow separation principle has been further evolved into an ingenious dual stage separation channel. This channel is eccentrically shaped so that different centrifugal forces operate in the two halves of the channel. In the first half platelets or buffy coat rich plasma are separated from the red cells, where in the second half the platelets or white cells are extracted from the plasma (Hester 1979). The dual stage separation channel is particularly suitable for the harvesting of highly purified platelets or white cell fractions.

A replica of the Cobe/IBM 2997 dual stage principle has been marketed by Dideco. The Vivacell BT 789C continuous flow blood cell separator was developed out of the BT 798 Viva plasma exchange unit. This machine displays the separation stages on a screen, but still requires the same degree of operator attention and adjusting action. So far, only few data have been published with respect to the efficiency of both BT 798 and 798C models.

Fenwal have developed a highly automated computer controlled apheresis machine, which for the processing of blood combines the circumferential and the axial separation principles (Buchholz et al 1982). The software is completely closed and consists of two bag-shaped asymmetrically segmented separation chambers in the centrifuge drum. The connections of the two chambers and the fixed exterior are via an Adams-type seal-less multilumen tube, which rotates in a skip rope fashion. This unique configuration seemingly defies the laws of physics as it spins at speeds of up to 1400 rpm without twisting or coiling, while blood and components pass through its five-lumen pathway. Blood flows into the first wedge-shaped separation chamber, where the plasma containing platelets and or granulocytes are separated from the red cells. The platelet rich plasma is then passed to the rectangular second separation chamber, where the cells are extracted from the plasma. The instrument can be used to harvest platelets, granulocytes or plasma from normal healthy donors. A programme for each type of collection procedure is stored in the solid state memory of the CS 3000, and can be operated both automatically and manually. The controlling microprocessor monitors the operation and the donor safety alarms in either mode of operation. The Fenwal CS 3000 is undoubtedly the easiest cell separator to operate because of its high degree of automation. As the separation and collection of components take place in the vertically positioned separation chambers within the centrifuge drum, the operator cannot see the product as it collects inside the centrifuge. A major disadvantage is the heavy weight of the instrument which limits mobility: a matter of some importance for bedside apheresis.

The first generation of this machine was not well adapted to therapeutic haemapheresis, but recent modifications have improved these functions.

Filtration principles

Based on the dialysis principle an alternative approach for therapeutic plasma exchange was developed in the 1970s using semiporous membranes (Solomon et al 1978). The primary aim has been the removal of protein bound pathogenic substances present in plasma. To achieve this purpose the membrane must be of such permeability as to allow the passage of the protein-bound pathogenic substances, while blocking the filtration of cellular elements. Both flat sheet membranes arranged as a sandwich and multiple tubulous membranes or hollow fibre systems have been used. For an optimal efficacy both in filtration capacity and biocompatibility, many variables need to be considered:
1. geometry of the pathway
2. membrane composition, structure and porosity
3. flow rate during the passage of the blood
4. transmembrane filtration pressure
5. total area of the blood-to-membrane exposure
6. sterilizability and release of toxic metabolites.

The configuration of both the sandwich and the hollow fibre systems permits a blood flow parallel to the membrane surface. The filtration of plasma therefore occurs perpendicularly through the membrane. The major efficacy factor is the sieving coefficient, the ratio of filtered material over the material present in the inflowing blood (Chmiel 1983). This efficacy factor is determined by the prefilter pressure, the pore size and the total filtration surface area. The hydrodynamic forces of the blood flow through the filter result in a transmembrane filtration pressure, which is highest at the inflow and lowest at the outflow part of the filter. Filtration efficacy therefore declines where simultaneously the blood viscosity increases. This automatically leads to a decrease in flow rate, resulting in a tendency of blood cells to pile up against the membrane. Convective forces towards the surface are encountered by an opposing fluid shear force. These shear forces may induce cell distortion and ultimate haemolysis. Depending on the polymers used, plasma protein molecules such as albumin may polarise at the membrane surface, affecting the plasma filtration flow. The semiporous membrane material must permit efficient plasma separation, while preventing cells from passing. The surface area must also be biocompatible to ensure minimal adverse effects on blood cells and proteins exposed to polymers. Additionaly it is required that there will be no toxic effects, no leaching of harmful substances or metabolites from the synthetic material and minimal complement activation. The materials used are cellulose di- and tri-acetate, polypropene and polypropylene, polyvinyl chloride derivatives, polyvinylidene fluoride, polyvinyl alcohol and copolymers of ethylene and vinyl alcohol.

The alcohols differ distinctly from the other synthetic polymers by their exclusive hydrophylic properties. These polymers are insolubilized by cross-linking and the material does not contain plasticisers or additives. Another distinct difference is in the possibility for steam sterilising the filters, where all other materials need either ethylene oxide or gamma irradiation treatment for sterilisation.

The standard pore sizes for primary plasma filtration membranes vary from 0.2 to 0.77 micrometers with effective surface areas ranging from 0.12 m^2 to 0.65 m^2 and perfusion volumes of 14–35 ml.

For therapeutic plasma exchange secondary filters used in a cascade system have been developed, with the aim of selectively removing specific protein-bound pathologic substances or macromolecules (Gregory et al 1984). The principles applied to this specific elimination of unwanted substances are manyfold and include ultrafiltration, cryogelation, adsorption and precipitation by chemical and physicochemical processes.

Ultrafiltration

Plasma collected by centrifugation or primary filtration may be passed over a secondary membrane. This provides a further option: the separation of albumin from the remaining plasma proteins, which include the large molecular substances such as IgG, IgA, IgM, immune complexes and lipid. The salvaged albumin is returned to the patient, thereby reducing the need for replacement. These secondary filters have a pore size of 0.06 micrometer and an effective surface area of $1.0–1.2 \text{ m}^2$. Depending on the pore size and surface area, further selective separation can be achieved, eliminating substances greater in molecular size than IgG such as IgM and immune complexes. This cascade principle allows selective removal of specific pathogenic substances although limiting the usefulness to only certain diseases. Currently a limited number of cascade filters are available such as Albusave

DT901 (Dideco), Plasmax QS-12-50 (Toray) and the Evaflux type 2A and 4A (Kuraray).

Cryogelation

Another option is the aggregation and removal of cryoglobulins, achieved by cooling at 4°C followed by filtration at a pore size of 0.1 micrometer (Abe et al 1983). This allows specific elimination of pathogenic cryoglobulins and immune complexes. A major problem, however, is the rapid clogging of the microporous membrane. Also cryogelation induces simultaneous depletion of normal cold insoluble globulins, such as fibronectin, fibrinogen and Factor VIII. Cryogelation chambers and filters for specific elimination of cryoglobulins are currently marketed by amongst others Cobe and Toray.

Adsorption

A number of affinity columns have been developed for the removal of pathogenic substances (Lysaght et al 1985). The principle is one of passing plasma through a column of an inert solid matrix to which an antibody is bound. Bound antibody will remove the corresponding antigen from the plasma and the effluent is reinfused into the patient. Depending on the type of adsorbent, a variety of matrixes can be used including sepharose, glass beads, silica, charcoal collodion and agarose. Most of these principles are currently under investigation. The field of immunoadsorption by affinity column technology is extremely promising and exciting. However, important potential problems are adsorptive capacity, the possibility for eluting either matrix or adsorbent into the patient's circulation, selection of optimal flow geometry, the stability of matrix-bound adsorbents and the ability to reuse the columns for the same patient. The affinity columns currently under testing are as follows.

1. Activated charcoal column (used for the in vitro extraction of bile acids)
2. DNA collodion charcoal column (for the specific immune adsorption and removal of single stranded DNA antibodies and immune complexes as circulating in for instance acute lupus glomerulonephritis)
3. Heparin agarose column (for the removal of cholesterol in homozygous familial hypercholesterolaemia. However, clinical experiments with heparin agarose affinity column plasma perfusion have led to serious reactions possibly due to activation of the alternate pathway of complement).
4. Anti LDL sepharose column (for the removal of low density lipoprotein including cholesterol in hyperlipidaemia).
5. A and B antigen columns (for effective removal of circulating high titre iso-agglutinins in for instance colon carcinoma patients and the removal of alloagglutinins in ABH incompatible bone marrow for transplantation.

These columns consist of synthetic sugar chains analogous to A and B blood group substance linked to a crystal silica bead).
6. Staphyllococcus protein A columns (have been used with acceptable efficacy in both haemoperfusion and plasma perfusion of patients with multiple myeloma, autoimmune haemolytic anaemia in chronic lymphocytic leukaemia, colonic carcinoma and for the release of blocked tumoricidal antibodies by adsorbing the binding agents).
7. Triptophane polyvinyl alcohol resin column (for the specific binding of anti-acetylcholinesterase receptor antibodies in myasthenia gravis).

Chemical and physico-chemical processes

On a research scale a variety of principles for precipitating specific pathogenic substances by chemical and physico-chemical principles such as enzymatic systems, electrophoretic and electrodialytic techniques have been tried (Pineda 1986). These techniques have not reached the clinic stage but may become an alternative approach to eliminating causative or enhancing coexistent pathogenic material in a number of defined diseases.

Equipment

Most machines developed for filtration apheresis are based on the existing haemodialysis technology. The equipment usually consists of a set of speed controlled roller pumps and built in microprocessors to monitor and control critical parameters such as blood flow rates, prefilter pressures, reinfusion rates, venous pressures and the detection of air. Increasingly, machines are equipped for double filtration techniques and allow the addition of cryogelation chambers kept at 4°C. For therapeutic plasma exchange the Japanese are well on their way to dominate both the hardware and disposables market. Among the machine manufacturers are Kawasumi, Nikiso, Kuraray and Toray all from Japan, and Cobe, Gambro, Dideco and Organon Teknika. Plasma filtration equipment is essentially simple, safe and easy to operate. The small size of most machines allows easy bedside manoeuvring.

For donor plasmapheresis by filtration only a few automated machines have been developed, sofar. Organon Teknika, Dideco and a Japanese company (Nipro) manufacture a filtration plasmapheresis system, consisting of a more or less automated machine and a software set which includes a hollow fibre filter. The synthetic semiporous membrane materials used are polypropene, polypropylene and cellulose acetate with pore sizes ranging from 0.55 to 0.65 μm and effective surface areas ranging from 0.07 to 0.5 m^2. The Organon Teknika machine differs in principle from the two other types, as it recirculates the blood collected after first filtration back over the filter while being mixed with freshly drawn donor blood. This is achieved by differentiating the speeds of the two blood pumps (Fig. 5.1).

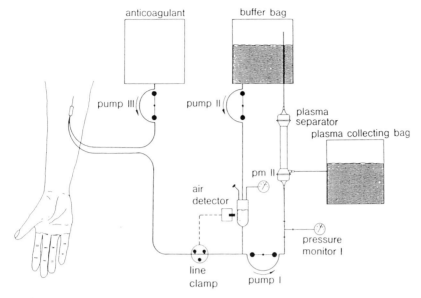

Fig. 5.1 Organon Teknika hollow fibre filtration plasmapheresis system (Phase 2).
Phase 1: Following filtration the red cells are collected in the buffer bag. Phase 2: The red cells are mixed with donor blood by differentiating the speed of pump I and pump II, and refiltered. Phase 3: The refiltered red cells are returned to the donor.

Table 5.1   Recommendations for starting a haemapheresis programme

To start a haemapheresis programme some recommendations may be helpful
1. Define purpose and need of the haemapheresis programme
   – is it donor defined?
   for supportive haemotherapy
   for plasma collection
   for both
   – is it therapeutic haemapheresis?
   – is it both donor and therapeutic haemapheresis?
2. Define frequency of use.
3. Define options for personnel
   training, expertise, continuing education
   technical and medical support.
4. Define location
   fixed site – bloodbank, hospital, other location
   mobility
   combined programme.
5. Define mode of financing
   equipment, disposables, replacement fluids,
   personnel.

When these fundamental questions have been answered the choice of machine will be further defined by the four major characteristics:
a. simplicity   – personnel, technical support, software availability
b. multipurpose – bloodbank or hospital setting
c. mobility   – need for bedside or mobile team situations
d. stability   – maintenance and technical support, power supply, spare parts.

A major disadvantage of donor plasmapheresis by filtration is the need for a constant blood flow rate in order to build up an adequate prefilter pressure which allows an optimal transmembrane pressure for efficient plasma filtration. This requires active participation of the donor and a continued alertness of the personnel. The combined centrifugation and flat membrane filtration principle as described above has so far been shown to be superior. This is not only because of the high degree of machine automation, but more importantly because of the elegant hydrodynamic principle applied.

Most filtration designs for therapeutic plasma exchange are based on the continuous flow principle, requiring two venepunctures. However, the donor plasma filtration machines all use a single needle discontinuous flow technique.

Selection of a machine

There is no simple answer to the question, 'Which is the best buy for a haemapheresis programme?' The answer will emerge as a consequence of considering a number of operational matters, as defined in Table 5.1.

OPTIONS FOR THE FUTURE

The developments in machine apheresis have been hitherto dominated by the need to support patient care. Both the techniques for collection of platelets and white cells from donors as well as therapeutic haemapheresis have developed rapidly and often in unforeseen directions. Anticipation of clinical demands for specific haemotherapy support have led to optimisation of the fundamental principles as developed some decades ago. For all these developments a more precise understanding of hydrodynamic aspects of cell separation for harvesting purified blood fractions in donor apheresis and a more precise conception of the pathophysiology of diseases is still needed.

For the future a further introduction of microprocessor control of the equipment will lead to increased safety and ease of processing. The user friendliness will improve so that more attention can be given to the donor or patient and operating stress will be much releaved.

There is a need for reducing the extracorporeal processing volume by miniaturizing the collection chambers. Here, alternative approaches to the separation of cells or plasma from donors, or the elimination of pathogenic substances from patients may lead to new designs and the introduction of revolutionary principles as presently under construction by HemaScience, Haemonetics and Sarns/3M.

The application of the plasma collection concept as developed by HemaScience for harvesting platelets in a closed haemapheresis system is not only exciting, but also opens opportunities to further exploration of cell purification technology. The present invention provides a method and

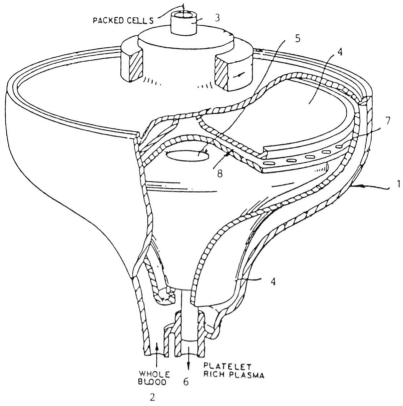

PACKED CELLS

WHOLE
BLOOD

PLATELET
RICH PLASMA

Fig. 5.2 The HemaScience blood collection and separation device. 1. Stationary housing. 2. Asymmetrically positioned whole blood inlet port. 3. Outlet for red cells. 4. Double walled rotor concentric with the housing. 5. Lengthwise passageway leading to, 6. Outlet port for platelet rich plasma, coaxial with the central axis. 7. Apertures in the outer wall of the rotor to allow red cell flow. 8. Red cell flow.

system which is effective for the separation of blood components, employing a small volume completely closed disposable system, in contrast to most currently employed open seal systems. This haemapheresis system and method comprises a stationary closed housing that has an inner concentric wall about a central axis (Fig. 5.2). The upper and lower ports communicate with the interior of the housing. Within the stationary housing is a double shell rotor concentrically mounted and rotatable about the central axis within the housing. There is a predetermined space between the outer rotor wall and the inner wall of the stationary housing, permitting blood to enter this housing cavity at its lower end and to rise. The ingenious part of this invention is in the design which allows blood to move through an aperture in the lower part of the rotor wall into a centrifugation gap defined by a concentric inner wall or core. While the blood advances upwards it is subjected to centrifugation. The residence time and rotational rate are selected so that near the top of the rotor heavier cellular matter such as erythrocytes are concentrated at the outer radial region and withdrawn through carefully positioned orifices in the wall that communicate with the upper outlet port in the housing. Lighter matter such as platelets move upwardly over the top of the core to a central orifice which passes downward along the central axis to a conical outlet. A differential flow impedence limits the upper blood flow in the gap between the rotor and the stationary housing. The passageway of preference therefore is the centrifugation gap, allowing continuous separation of the majority of the input whole blood into the desired fractions. A magnetic drive external to the housing couples to an internal magnetic element mounted to the upper part of the rotor so as to achieve the needed rotational velocity. The design is oval shaped and in contrast to the conventional bowls used for cell separation is positioned upside down.

The principle described is of particular applicability for the separation

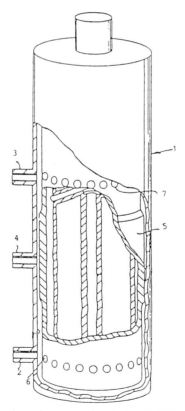

Fig. 5.3 The HemaScience secondary separation device. 1. Stationary housing. 2. Inlet port for platelet rich plasma. 3. Outlet port for platelet concentrate. 4. Inlet port for plasma or saline. 5. Double walled rotor as a modified circular cylinder. 6. Inlet apertures for input of platelet rich plasma into the centrifugation gap region. 7. Outlet apertures for platelet concentrate, in communication with the outlet port 3.

of the packed red cells from the platelet rich plasma portion of whole blood. However, it can also be employed for the collection of granulocytes, lymphocytes and neocytes. Another part of the invention is a membrane filtration device, essentially similar to the plasmapheresis system, which in conjunction with the first separator allows continuous extraction of red cells and plasma for return to the donor, while platelet concentrate is collected separately. This membrane filtration device also has an interior spinner within a stationary housing. The bowl-shaped prototype has been developed into a cylindrical biologically closed system for separating lighter and heavier constituents from an input blood flow. This new design compares to the Autopheresis-C plasmacell, but the difference is in the configuration of the inner rotating part (Fig. 5.3). The two parts of this invention can be assembled in such a way that plasma collected by filtration in the second part can be returned with the red cells to the donor. Optionally a fraction of the plasma can be pumped back to the cell separator, to help elutriate the platelets from the blood (Fig. 5.4). The device is also driven by an external magnetic drive. The invention is designed as a discontinuous flow system. It is claimed to be biologically closed and to be run at low cost.

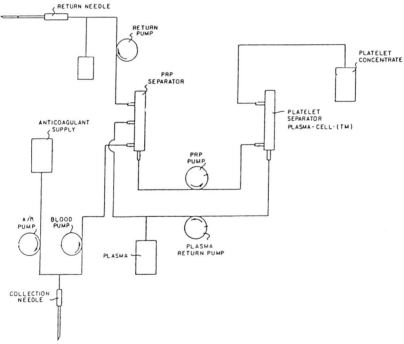

Fig. 5.4 The HemaScience biological closed disposable system composed of the primary PRP separator and the secondary platelet concentrate separator for blood processing. The original system is a two needle set-up, where blood is separated into PRP and red cells by centrifugation. In the secondary platelet separator the plasma is separated from the platelets by elutriative centrifugation. Optionally a fraction of the plasma can be pumped back to the primary cell separator to help elutriate the platelet rich plasma from the blood.

Haemonetics has developed a highly automated small portable version of the PCS. The grenade shaped separation chamber has been redesigned to optimise the hydrodynamics and to miniaturize the extracorporeal volume. The weak point of the bowl, the rotating seal, has been further developed by the application of a shrink lap on the head of the bowl. This is claimed to guarantee absolute closure of the system. The machine weighs only 15 kg and can be run at low cost in a mobile team setting.

In 1983 Sarns/3M and Millipore Inc. agreed to join forces and develop new approaches to machine apheresis. The result has been the creation of an attractive and innovative alternative in membrane plasmapheresis technology. The core of the system is a highly sophisticated separation module which incorporates a polyvinylidene fluoride microporous membrane developed by Millipore Inc. The highly automated microprocessor controlled system consists of four components (Fig. 5.5): a miniature sized microporous membrane separation module, a colour-coded polyvinylchloride

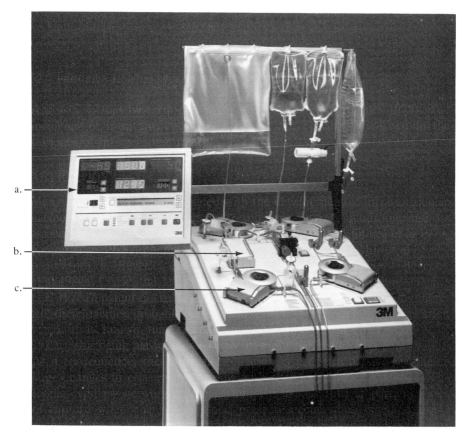

Fig. 5.5 The Sarns Therapeutic Apheresis System. a. Control panel. b. Miniature microporous membrane separation module. c. Portable pump console.

tubeset, a small portable pumpconsole and a control panel mounted on an adjustable arm. The separation module contains alternating layers of biocompatible polyvinylidene fluoride microporous membranes and polycarbonate membrane spacers, which create separate channels for blood and plasma flows that closely resemble pre-capillary circulation. Plasma removal efficiency, at rates up to 40 ml per minute, average 60% in this continuous flow process. The control panel allows the operator to transmit patient data to the microprocessor, prime the system automatically, stop and easily restart the plasma separation process and monitor the progress of the therapeutic plasma exchange procedure. The system continuously monitors transmembrane pressures and adjusts plasma flow to prevent haemolysis.

These developments reflect a major endeavour in innovating machine haemapheresis by exploring all possible options. Safety, purity, potency and clinical efficacy are of paramount importance for the future developments in this field including the exciting options for more specific manipulative technologies such as elutriation, ultrafiltration, selective immunoadsorption and physicochemical plasmaprotein separation systems.

REFERENCES

Abe Y, Smith J W, Malchesky P S, Nosé Y 1983 Cryofiltration: Development and current status. Plasma Therapy Transfusion Technology 4: 405–414
Abel J J, Rowntree L G, Turner B B, 1914 Plasma removal with return of corpuscles (plasmapheresis). Journal of Pharmacology and Experimental Therapeutics: Baltimore 5: 625–641
Buchholz D H, Porten J H, Menitove J E, et al 1982 Description and use of the CS-3000 blood cell separator for single donor platelet collection Transfusion 23: 190–196
Chmiel H 1983 The effects of pressure, flow conditions and surface composition on the filtration properties of plasma separation modules. Plasma Therapy and Transfusion Technology 4: 387–396
Derksen R H W M 1983 Plasma exchange in human disease. Academic Thesis University of Utrecht, Utrecht
Djerassi I, Kim J S, Mitrakul C, Suvansri U, Ciesielka W 1970 Filtration leukapheresis for separation and concentration of transfusable amounts of normal human granulocytes. Journal of Medicine (Basel), 1: 358–364
van Edc H 1985 De surge V50 aferese machine: Een vergelijkend onderzoek met oude en nieuwe programma's naar de opbrengst van plaatjesconcentraat en de contaminatie met witte bloedcellen. Project report Red Cross Blood Bank, Groningen-Drenthe, Groningen
Elias M, Oenema B, Scholten J T, Das P C, Smit Sibinga C Th 1985 Surge pump platelet apheresis: A method for effective depletion of white cells from machine-collected single donor platelets. Plasma Therapy Transfusion Technology 6: 381–386
Freireich E J, Judson G, Levin R H 1965 Separation and collection of leucocytes. Cancer Research 25: 1516–1520
Gregory M C, Shettigar U R, Kolff W J 1984 Theoretical value of cascade plasmapheresis. Plasma Therapy Transfusion Technology 5: 517–529
Hester J P 1979 Variable anti-coagulant (AC) flow rates for plateletpheresis in the dual stage disposable channel. Blood 54: (Suppl. 1) 124[a] (abstract 303)
Hester J P, Kellogg R M, Mulzet A P, Kruger V R, McCredie K P, Freireich E J 1979 Principles of blood separation and component extraction in a disposable continuous-flow single-stage channel. Blood 54: 254–268
Huestis D W, Bove J R, Bush S 1981 Practical Blood Transfusion pp 351–354 Brown and Company 3rd edition, Boston

Latham Jr A, Kingsley G F 1975 Cell separator design considerations. In Leucocytes: separation, collection and transfusion, Goldman J M, Lowenthal R M, Eds. Academic Press, London, New York, San Francisco pp 203–207

Lysaght M J, Samtleben W, Schmidt B, Gurland H J 1985 In Therapeutic Hemapheresis Vol. I: MacPherson J L, Kasprisin, Eds. Boca Raton, FL: CRC Press, pp 149–168

Pineda A A 1986 Future directions of apheresis. In Therapeutic Hemapheresis, Valbonesi M, Pineda A A, Biggs J C, Eds. Milan: Wichtig Editore, pp 187–194

Pineda A A, Taswell H F 1981 Selective plasma component removal: Alternatives to plasma exchange. Artificial Organs 5: 234–240

Schoendorfer D W, Hansen L E, Kennedy D M 1983 The surge technique: A method to increase purity of platelet concentrates obtained by centrifugal apheresis. Transfusion 23: 182–189

Smit Sibinga C Th 1986 Apheresis machines and techniques. In Therapeutic Hemapheresis, Valbonesi M, Pineda A A, Biggs J C, Eds. Milan: Wichtig Editore, pp 1–8

Solomon B A, Castino F, Lysaght M J, Colton C K, Friedman L I 1978 Continuous flow membrane filtration of plasma from whole blood. Transactions – American Society for Artificial Internal Organs 24:21

Tullis J L, Surgenor D M, Tinch R J et al 1956 New principle of closed system centrifugation. Science 124: 792–797

Tullis J L, Tinch R J, Bandanza P et al 1971 Plateletapheresis in a disposable system. Transfusion 11: 368–377

Leucocyte-depleted blood components

INTRODUCTION

All standard blood components are contaminated with leucocytes, which may cause important transfusion complications. Foreign leucocytes can stimulate the production of alloantibodies directed against both HLA and leucocyte-specific antigens (Barton 1981, Décary et al 1984, De Rie et al 1985) which in turn can be the cause of the febrile transfusion reactions (Payne 1957, Brittingham & Chaplin 1957), refractoriness to platelet transfusions (Herzig et al 1975, Eernisse & Brand 1981) and rejection of transplants (Kissmeyer-Nielsen et al 1966). Transfused leucocytes may determine graft versus-host disease in patients with congenital or acquired severe immunodeficiency (Hathaway et al 1967, Ford et al 1976). Moreover, some viruses, such as cytomegalovirus (CMV), can be transmitted by leucocytes (Rinaldo et al 1977, Schrier et al 1985, Verdonck et al 1985). Finally, there is increasing in vitro and in vivo evidence that blood transfusion has an immunodepressive effect and this also seems to be due, at least in some conditions, to transfused leucocytes: depressed NK cell function (Gascòn et al 1984, Kaplan et al 1984, Sirchia et al 1986), T lymphocyte subset abnormalities (Kaplan et al 1984, Neri et al 1984, Grady et al 1985, De Martino et al 1985, Sirchia et al 1986a), and decreased response of T cells to mitogens (Munn et al 1981, De Martino et al 1985) have been reported. While some of the above in vitro abnormalities can be induced by concomitant factors, blood transfusion also has immunodepressive effects in vivo. Transfusions determine an increased graft survival in renal transplant patients (Opelz et al 1973, Opelz 1985) and have been suspected of influencing negatively both patient survival and frequency of tumor recurrences in patients with colorectal, breast and lung cancer (Burrows & Tartter 1982, Blumberg et al 1985, Foster et al 1985, Hyman et al 1985). Recently, blood transfusion has been reported to cause CMV infection in previously CMV-infected patients through reactivation of endogenous CMV, probably due to a transient immunodepressive effect rather than through reinfection with an exogenous strain of CMV (Adler et al 1985).

All these findings suggest that blood transfusion elicits an immuno-depressive effect through the transmission of some viruses and/or the introduction into the recipient of some alloantigens. For immune depression towards the transplanted kidney, at least, there is evidence that these alloantigens are present on transfused leucocytes. In fact, leucocyte-free blood transfusions are not capable of determining the favourable effect on kidney graft survival known as the 'transfusion effect' (Persijn et al 1979); moreover if the number of mononuclear cells in the transfused blood is lowered below a certain limit, the resulting 'transfusion effect' is less than that obtained with standard blood transfusions, so that the survival and function of the transplanted kidney become intermediate between those of untransfused subjects and those of patients given standard blood transfusions (Sirchia et al 1982a).

CLINICAL INDICATIONS FOR LEUCOCYTE-DEPLETED RED CELL UNITS

Prevention of the nonhaemolytic febrile transfusion reaction

So far leucocyte-depleted red cells have been mainly used to prevent the occurrence of the nonhaemolytic febrile transfusion reaction (NHFTR) in patients with antileucocyte antibodies. The maximum number of contaminating leucocytes that these patients can tolerate without developing a reaction varies and probably depends on many factors, such as the type and strength of the antibodies present in the patient's serum, the type of white blood cells contained in the blood unit and the rate at which the blood is transfused. Perkins et al (1966) first suggested that some patients may respond with fever to the administration of as few as 250×10^6 leucocytes, whereas others tolerate without fever as many as 2500×10^6 leucocytes which is the average number contained in a standard blood unit. Although an exhaustive investigation of this problem has not been done, experience shows that blood units containing less than 250×10^6 leucocytes are capable of preventing almost all the reactions caused by leucocytes even in multitransfused highly immunized patients, and units containing $790 \pm 230 \times 10^6$ leucocytes decrease by half the incidence of NHFTR (Lidén & Hildén 1982). Therefore, although a satisfactory definition of leucocyte-*poor* red cells is lacking, for practical purposes the choice is between a leucocyte-poor (averaging 1000×10^6 leucocytes/unit) and -*very poor* (less than 250×10^6/unit) blood product depending on the level of reaction of the patient.

Prevention of antileucocyte antibody production

A second indication for leucocyte-depleted red cells is to reduce the risk of sensitizing the recipient to leucocyte antigens. In fact, there is still no clear demonstration that this is possible, but evidence is growing that the administration of red cell units containing no detectable leucocytes is capable of preventing or delaying the production of antileucocyte antibodies in previously nonstimulated subjects (Sirchia et al 1986). The use of leucocyte-*free* red cells may then be of great value in some categories of patients such as prospective organ transplant recipients (to avoid the production of broad-spectrum lymphocytotoxic antibodies that not only make it difficult to find a compatible donor (Bollinger et al 1982) but also seem to have a negative effect on graft survival (Opelz 1985) or in prospective recipients of long-term transfusion support. The administration of leucocyte-free red cell and platelet concentrates to acute leukaemia patients from the beginning of treatment could represent a step forward in the transfusion treatment of these patients. In fact about half of them develop anti-HLA antibodies and become refractory to random platelet transfusions (Schiffer et al 1976, Howard & Perkins 1978). To overcome this life-threatening complication, single-donor, HLA-compatible platelets can be used (Yankee et al 1969, Duquesnoy et al 1977), but this requires a huge organizational effort and is not always effective in the long term even if HLA-compatible donors can be found. Another approach for these immunized patients is to resort to platelet autotransfusion (Schiffer et al 1978): for patients who produce antibodies during induction chemotherapy, autologous platelets are collected during remission and stored frozen to be used when refractoriness to homologous platelets occurs. This type of programme, however, is expensive and not feasible in all patients. The combination of prevention of antibody formation with the above two procedures is expected to improve the quality of treatment given to these patients. Prospective trials are in progress in Europe (Rebulla & Sirchia 1985, Brand 1985, Koerner & Kubanek 1987) and the USA (Sniecinski 1986) with the aim of determining whether transfusing acute leukaemia patients with leucocyte-free red cell and platelet concentrates from the very onset of the disease is capable of preventing the occurrence of antileucocyte antibodies and refractoriness to platelet transfusions. These clinical investigations are based on the observation that in children with thalassaemia major transfused every three to four weeks for a median of 50 times the transfusion of packed red cells made leucocyte-free by filtration from the beginning of transfusion treatment did not determine the occurrence of antileucocyte antibodies, whereas 70% of similar patients given leucocyte-poor red cell units developed such alloantibodies (Sirchia et al 1982b, 1986).

The definition of leucocyte-free red cell and platelet concentrates requires some comments. 'Free' in this context is used to indicate 'free of detectable leucocytes' by conventional techniques; this does not mean tht cell concentrates do not contain a few thousand leucocytes (Vakkila & Myllylä 1986) or fragments of leucocytes and platelets or antigens shed by their membranes. That this is the case was in fact shown by Engelfriet et al (1975) in animal experiments and more recently by Vos et al (1987) by using a radioimmunoassay for the detection of the platelet glycoprotein complex IIb–IIIa. This probably explains why leucocyte-free red cell units are apparently not capable of preventing the occurrence of antileucocyte antibodies in previously stimulated recipients (Scornik et al 1984) or abnormalities of some in vitro immunological tests even in previously nonstimulated multitransfused patients (Sirchia et al 1986).

CRITERIA FOR EVALUATING METHODS OF LEUCOCYTE DEPLETION

In vitro parameters

Assuming that the procedure does not reduce the safety and efficacy of the product, a reasonable set of data that can be used in the Transfusion Centre to evaluate a procedure of leucocyte depletion is the following:
Red cell recovery, determined by evaluating the packed red cell volume in the unit before and after the leucocyte-depleting treatment.
Number and type of leucocytes, determined before and after the leucocyte-depleting treatment by an automatic cell counter. When the number of contaminating leucocytes is low, a manual count can be more accurate (Milner et al 1982); it is therefore advisable after processing to evaluate the number of residual leucocytes microscopically in a counting chamber, after 1:10 dilution of a thoroughly mixed blood sample with Turk's solution.

In vivo parameters

If the purpose is to prepare leucocyte-poor red cell units to prevent NHFTR, the following in vivo parameters can be used (Schned & Silver 1981):

$$\text{Transfusion reaction rate (TRR)} = \frac{\text{No. of transfusions complicated by NHFTR}}{\text{No. of transfusions}} \times 100$$

$$\text{Patient reaction rate (PRR)} = \frac{\text{No. of patients presenting NHFTR}}{\text{No. of patients transfused}} \times 100$$

If the purpose is to prepare leucocyte-free red cell (or platelet) concentrates to avoid sensitization to leucocyte antigens, the latter two parameters should be substituted by monitoring the recipient for antileucocyte antibodies.

In the evaluation of a leucocyte depletion method other characteristics must be considered, primarily its reproducibility and cost-effectiveness, including its difficulty, the time needed for its completion and the shelf life of the product. Procedures requiring a unit of blood to be entered, i.e. open system processing, reduce the shelf life of the product to 24 h and can result in blood wastage if the transfusion is delayed or cancelled.

METHODS FOR THE PREPARATION OF LEUCOCYTE-POOR AND -FREE RED CELL (AND PLATELET) CONCENTRATES

As soon as it was shown that transfused leucocytes, particularly granulo-cytes (Perkins et al 1966), are the main cause of the NHFTR (Payne 1957, Brittingham & Chaplin 1957) attempts were started to prepare a new blood component, i.e. leucocyte-poor red cells for transfusion. Over a period of about 30 years many techniques have been developed (see Polesky 1977, Meryman et al 1980, Hughes & Brozović 1982, Parravicini et al 1983, Wenz 1986 for references), but the ideal method is still lacking even though much progress has been made.

Although many methodological variations exist, leucocyte depletion of red cells is currently obtained by 5 basic techniques: differential centrifu-gation, sedimentation, cell washing, freezing and thawing, and filtration. The procedures reported so far, moreover, can be divided into those that, because of the manoeuvres required, must be carried out in the transfusion centre and those that can be performed in the ward at the bedside. The effectiveness of the principal procedures is summarized in the Appendix.

Methods to be used in the transfusion centre

Differential centrifugation

This is perhaps the simplest and most frequently used technique for the preparation of leucocyte-poor red cells. When the blood bag is centrifuged, due to their different sedimentation coefficients, lymphocytes and platelets tend to collect above the packed volume of erythrocytes forming the 'buffy coat', whereas most granulocytes are found in the upper portion of the red cell layer. If this portion of red cells is removed together with the buffy coat, an acceptable leucocyte-poor red cell concentrate can be obtained. Expression of the buffy coat can be facilitated by the application of a stomach clamp on the blood bag at the desired level to separate the buffy coat from the red cell layer (Prins et al 1980). The major disadvantages of this procedure are the high red cell loss and the poor reproducibility. More-over, if a satellite bag is not used to transfer the buffy coat, the technique's shortcomings also include open system processing. In an attempt to improve these results various modifications of the basic technique have been described, including inverted centrifugation, double centrifugation, upright centrifugation of red cells diluted with saline, but with the exception of the last modification, they do not improve the original procedure significantly (Meryman et al 1980). Schneider & Stützle (1979) described a method in which the buffy coat formed during centrifugation of units preincubated at 37°C for 60 min is removed with a special separation apparatus (Biotest, FRG). The efficacy of this method in removing leucocytes and platelets has been confirmed by Koerner & Stampe (1982) and by Shimizu et al (1986); however 140 min are required to perform this technique. All in all, leucocyte-poor red cell units prepared by simply removing the buffy coat after centrifugation can still be considered a valid blood product (Menitove et al 1982, Rock et al 1984), capable of reducing the incidence of NHFTR by some 50% in a standard clinical setting (Liéden & Hildén 1982).

Sedimentation

If agents that increase the erythrocyte sedimentation rate, such as dextran solutions, are added to the blood and this is allowed to sediment, approximately 80% of the leucocytes can be removed by eliminating the supernatant fluid and the buffy coat. If the blood is processed a second time, 98% of the leucocytes can be removed with a negligible red cell loss (Chaplin et al 1959). In our laboratory, a double dextran sedimentation has been used for years for the preparation of leucocyte-very poor red cells for the transfusion treatment of highly immunized patients: in fact, this procedure allows us to obtain red cell units containing less than 50×10^6 leucocytes in 97% of treated standard units with a median red cell loss of 14% (Sirchia et al 1980). The procedure however is cumbersome, and requires open system processing. Today it has no place in the transfusion centre.

Cell washing

Whereas manual washing of a red cell unit is too impractical to be proposed for the preparation of leucocyte-poor red cells, even though the minimum of 70% leucocyte removal with 70% red cell recovery required by the Standards of the American Association of Blood Banks (Schmidt 1984) can be reached (Polesky et al 1973), automated red cell washing procedures by cell separators are still widely used. The effectiveness of white cell removal by automated cell washing depends on a number of variables, among which the most important are the number of washing cycles and the amount of red cell loss that is acceptable (Wenz 1986). In experienced centres leucocyte removal is 85–90% with a red cell loss of about 15% (Wooten 1976, Bryant et al 1978, Uda et al 1984, Lichtiger at al 1984). The main disadvantages of this technique are the high cost, the dependence on a machine and its disposables, and the 24 h expiry date of the product due to an open system of processing. We agree with Menitove et al (1982) that the use of machine-washed red cells should be limited to special cases. Among these are patients who experience reactions to plasma constituents; in these patients automated washing, by removing over 99% of the plasma proteins present in the unit (Wooten 1976), can prevent the transfusion reaction in almost all cases.

Freezing and thawing

Freeze-thaw and deglycerolization of red blood cells by automated cell washers remove plasma, platelets and leucocytes effectively by combining washing with cell fragmentation. Under the usual blood bank conditions of red cell freezing, be it the 'low glycerol' or the 'high glycerol' technique, leucocytes are poorly cryoprotected and most of them become fragmented on thawing and are removed by subsequent washing. The drawback of this procedure is its high cost. It is therefore not cost-effective for the preparation of leucocyte-poor red cells (Chaplin 1982) and cannot be recommended for the preparation of leucocyte-free red cells. Red cell units frozen with the low glycerol technique have in fact been shown to be associated with the production of antileucocyte antibodies in the recipient (Amer et al 1980, Minchinton et al 1980) and this is also so for red cells frozen with the high glycerol technique (Polesky 1977, Perkins 1977). The results obtained with this latter procedure vary considerably from author to author. In our laboratory, by using Valeri's procedure that processes red cells in the primary bag (Valeri et al 1981), we found that about 95% of leucocytes can be removed, so that residual leucocytes are 60×10^6/unit (median value). Leucocyte-very poor red cells have also been obtained by addition and removal of glycerol without freezing and thawing the blood unit (Crowley & Valeri 1974a, Kurtz et al 1981). The results of all these procedures are no better than those obtained by the simpler and less expensive procedures of blood filtration.

Filtration

In 1962 Greenwalt et al observed that the majority of granulocytes were removed from heparinized blood by a nylon filter. The need to collect the blood into an anticoagulant that limits storage to 48 h, the low red cell recovery, the use of open system processing and the ineffectiveness of the filter in removing lymphocytes were the main causes of the scarce attention given to this observation. Ten years later, Diepenhorst et al (1972) in Amsterdam developed a filter containing cotton wool that proved highly effective in depleting red cells of leucocytes and in preventing the occurrence of NHFTR (Diepenhorst & Engelfriet 1975). In the second half of the 70s, two kinds of filters were made commercially available for the preparation of leucocyte-poor red cells in the transfusion centre: Imugard ® IG-500 (Terumo, Japan) produced a column filter containing 22 g of a cotton wool obtained from 'Gossypium barbadense', and Erypur ® (Organon Teknika, The Netherlands) containing 55 g of cellulose acetate. In our opinion, the above filters constituted a major step forward in the preparation of leucocyte-depleted red cells. In fact, not only did they allow leucocyte-very poor red cells to be prepared simply and effectively at reasonable cost, but they made feasible the preparation of leucocyte-free red cell units for transfusion. We found (Sirchia et al 1982b) that with some simple precautions Erypur and Imugard IG-500 allowed the preparation of leucocyte-free red cell concentrates in 62% and 30% of processed standard units respectively, and in no case did the number of residual leucocytes

Table 6.1   In vitro effectiveness of Erypur and Imugard filtration, followed by light centrifugation and removal of the supernatant fluid (from Sirchia et al 1982b).

	Parameters					
				Leucocyte contamination/unit		
Procedures	Buffy coat in the filtered PRC[1] units	Filtered PRC units (No.)	Red cell recovery (%)	no detectable leucocytes	≤ 50 million	> 50 million
Filtration through Erypur filters	absent	266	93[2] (92–94)[3]	96[4]	4	0
	present	51	93 (91–94)	62	38	0
Filtration through Imugard filters[5]	absent	100	86 (85–87)	65	35	0
	present	100	87 (86– 88)	30	70	0

[1] Packed red cells 2–5 days old
[2] Median
[3] 95% confidence limits
[4] Percent of filtered PRC units
[5] Performed at about 10°C

exceed 50×10^6 (Table 6.1). They appeared therefore particularly suitable for those transfusion centres that have to provide blood for highly immunized multitransfused patients. There are several differences between the cotton wool and cellulose acetate filters. The residual leucocyte content is composed of both granulocytes and lymphocytes when Imugard is used, whereas almost only lymphocytes are present after Erypur filtration (Kikugawa & Minoshima 1978, Sirchia et al 1980). Imugard adsorbs a mean of 2400×10^6 leucocytes, which is the average number of leucocytes present in a standard unit of blood; Erypur adsorbs an average of 5200×10^6 leucocytes per filter (Reesink et al 1982).

In 1983 we reported that leucocyte-free platelet concentrates could be prepared by filtration of standard platelet concentrates through Imugard IG-500 (Sirchia et al 1983) (Table 6.2). The platelet loss was about 10% and filtered platelets were fully capable of correcting the bleeding time in thrombocytopenic patients. This observation, subsequently confirmed by many groups (Sniecinski et al 1986, Högman 1986, Sintnicolaas 1986, Hewson et al 1986, Masse et al 1986, Myllylä et al 1986, Andreu et al 1986, Koerner & Kubanek 1987), led to the previously mentioned clinical investigations on the prevention of refractoriness to platelet transfusion in acute leukaemia by transfusing patients from the beginning of treatment with leucocyte-free red cell and platelet concentrates. Similar investigations performed in recent years (Eernisse & Brand 1981, Robinson 1984, Murphy et al 1986) gave promising results, in spite of the fact that they all used not leucocyte-free but leucocyte-poor blood products; in fact they indicated that transfusion

Table 6.2 In vitro effectiveness of Imugard filtration for the preparation of leucocyte-free platelet concentrates from random or apheresis platelet concentrates (from Sirchia et al 1983).

Platelet concentrates		Before filtration		After filtration			
					Leucocyte contamination		
Type	No.	Number of platelets ($\times 10^{11}$)	Number of leucocytes ($\times 10^6$)	Platelet recovery (%)	no detectable leucocytes	$\leqslant 10$ million	> 10 million
Pool of eight random concentrates	45	5.5[1] (4.6–5.9)[2]	520 (390–660)	91 (88–95)	85[3]	12.5	2.5
Plateletpheresis (IBM 2997 dual-stage)	14	3.9 (3.3–4.7)	78 (40–165)	93 (84–100)	100	0	0
Plateletpheresis (Haemonetics Model 30 or Dideco Progress)	20[4]	3.1 (2.4–3.5)	376 (152–848)	95 (89–100)	75	25	0

[1] Median
[2] 95% confidence limits
[3] Percent of processed units
[4] Units centrifuged before filtration at 200 g for 10 min to remove most leucocytes

of patients with leucocyte-poor red cell and platelet concentrates reduced the incidence of alloimmunization in comparison with control patients treated with conventional blood components. A similar difference was also found by Schiffer et al (1983), but in this case it was not significant. These experiences suggest that, using leucocyte-free blood components, prevention of refractoriness to platelet transfusion in cancer patients may become a reality, and this is in fact supported by preliminary data recently reported by Sniecinski & O'Donnell (1986).

In spite of the many advantages, Erypur and Imugard filtration has distinct drawbacks. The rate at which leucocytes are removed depends on the anticoagulant used (Feng et al 1984) and on the temperature at which the procedure is carried out (Diepenhorst et al 1972, Kikugawa & Minoshima 1978, Sirchia et al 1982b). Both filters require open system processing and the average time needed for completing the procedure is 30–40 min (Reesink et al 1982, Lichtiger et al 1984); the semi automation made available for Erypur filtration (Prins et al 1978) has partly improved the situation. Even though new devices are still being produced to improve the preparation of leucocyte-depleted red cell units in the transfusion centre (Lovric et al 1981, Leng et al 1984) we have become progressively convinced that the real solution to the problems connected with the preparation of leucocyte-depleted red cells could be a filter used in the ward at the bedside.

Methods that can be used at the bedside

In 1980, Wenz et al (1980b) reported that substantial leucocyte removal could be achieved at the bedside by substituting the conventional blood administration filter of 170 μ with Ultipor® SQ40S (Pall Biomedicals, USA), a screen filter devised to retain microaggregates larger than 40 μ. The same group (Wenz et al 1980b, Wenz 1983) found that the effectiveness of leucocyte removal by Ultipor SQ40S increased if blood units stored for at least 3 weeks were centrifuged at high speed before filtration. Residual leucocytes were mainly lymphocytes, which could explain why the TRR of blood administered by this 'Spin and Filter' (SF) procedure was about one third that recorded with buffy coat-depleted red cell transfusions (Schned & Silver 1981). Centrifugation prior to filtration had the effect of increasing the number and size of microaggregates (Solis & Gibbs 1972) that in unprocessed blood units form spontaneously as a function of storage time due to the aggregation of degenerated leucocytes, platelets and fibrin (Swank 1961, McNamara et al 1971, Solis et al 1974). The effectiveness of SF, however, was limited when fresh blood units were processed. This problem was partly overcome by refrigerating for at least 3 h the centrifuged blood bag before filtration (Parravicini et al 1984). Refrigeration increases coalescence of microaggregates sedimented by centrifugation, with a resultant decrease in their fragility and an increase in their removal rate by the filter. This 'Spin Cool and Filter' (SCF) technique is less influenced by the unit's storage age, being effective also with 4 days old blood units, and consistently yields a product containing less than 500×10^6 leucocytes. In comparative studies, the SCF technique proved to be more effective than the SF procedure (Table 6.3).

Incidentally, SCF is capable of improving also the performance of Imugard filtration: the number of leucocyte-free red cell units obtained doubles if the blood bag is centrifuged and cooled before filtration through Imugard (Parravicini et al 1983).

Several unique advantages are offered by filtration through Ultipor

Table 6.3   Leucocyte removal and red cell recovery in standard packed red cell units processed through Ultipor SQ40S by Spin and Filter or Spin, Cool and Filter techniques (from Parravicini et al 1984).

Procedure	Processed PRC[1] units (No.)	Red cell recovery (%)	Leucocyte removal (%)	Residual leucocytes ($\times 10^6$)
Spin and filter	40	90.3[2] (83–97)[3]	71 (70–83)	920 (150–1400)
Spin, Cool and Filter	40	92.7 (82–98)	84.4 (82–92)	360 (110–1100)

[1] Packed red cells 4–9 days old
[2] Median
[3] Range

SQ40S for the preparation of leucocyte-poor red cells. The procedure becomes an open one at the time of administration and therefore does not reduce the product's shelf life nor does it cause blood wastage when the transfusion is delayed or cancelled. The red cell loss is minimal, averaging less than 10% of the original red cell mass (Wenz 1983, Parravicini et al 1984), and decreases if more than one unit is administered through a single filter; this on the other hand does not reduce the effectiveness of leucocyte removal for at least 3 units of blood and allows a further reduction of the already reasonable costs. Because of these major advantages some authorities recommend the use of microaggregate filters at the bedside as a first choice to produce leucocyte-poor red cells (Hughes & Brozović 1982, Mijović et al 1983, Meryman & Hornblower 1986), especially Ultipor with SCF (Meryman & Hornblower 1986). Units of blood which are not depleted of platelets prior to storage form microaggregates more avidly than those rendered platelet-poor (Reynolds & Simon 1980), but also these units allow a leucocyte deprivation of at least 70% by the SCF technique (Wenz 1986). Finally, better results can be obtained with this technique if the blood bag is handled carefully, so as not to disrupt the buffy coat, and infusion of the buffy coat is prevented by interrupting the transfusion at the appropriate time.

One disadvantage of the SCF technique through Ultipor SQ40S is that leucocyte-free red cell units cannot be obtained, so that NHFTR can occur in highly immunized patients if infusion of the buffy coat is not prevented. Moreover, blood collected in ACD, by decreasing pH, reduces platelet aggregation (Solis et al 1974) and consequently gives results that are less satisfactory than those obtained with blood collected in CPD. Finally, units preserved in mannitol-containing solutions do not form aggregates of sufficient size and composition to render the product leucocyte-poor by SCF through Ultipor SQ40S until the units have been stored at $+4°C$ for at least 2 weeks (Huang et al 1985, Wenz 1986). Other types of filters for microaggregates, i.e. depth (adsorption) filters and filters combining screening and adsorption, have been used to prepare leucocyte-poor red cells (Hurley et al 1978, Treleaven et al 1982, Wenz 1983, Parravicini et al 1983, Mijović et al 1983, Wenz & Apuzzo 1987). Unlike screen filters, which act simply by a sieving mechanism, depth filters act by binding different types of particulates according to the material used for their makeup (Lowe 1981). The main disadvantages of depth filters are a lower red cell recovery and long blood administration time (Cullen & Ferrara 1974, Parravicini et al 1983, Wenz 1983).

In order to evaluate the feasibility of SCF through Ultipor SQ40S in clinical practice, in 1985 we performed a prospective investigation on 81 thalassaemic patients who have been given transfusion treatment at our centre for a number of years (75 from 1980 and 6 others from 1981–83) (Parravicini et al 1987). In 1979, 35 of these patients had been diagnosed as having frequent NHFTR (defined as an increase in temperature of at least 1°C occurring during or within 8 h of transfusion in a previously afebrile patient, with no other apparent clinical cause for reaction) and/or severe arthralgias occurring during or just after the transfusion of standard packed red cells. All these 'more reactive' patients had lymphocytotoxic antibodies in their serum. They were treated thereafter with leucocyte-poor red cell units (prepared by double centrifugation in 1980–1982, then by Imugard filtration up to May 1985), whereas the remaining patients received standard or buffycoat depleted red cell units up to the beginning of the study. By this time all 81 thalassaemia patients were given standard packed red cell units made leucocyte-poor by SCF through Ultipor SQ40S. Two medical students at the transfusion centre collaborated with the nurses in informing the patients and their parents about the advantages of this procedure and in training them to discontinue the transfusion when the red cell layer, measured by a ruler at the outport of the bag, reached a height of 25 mm, so as to avoid infusion of the buffy coat. The evaluation of this procedure in vitro showed that Ultipor SQ40S halved leucocyte contamination of red cells in comparison to the standard 170 μ filter (Table 6.4). The results of the in vivo study are depicted in Figure 6.1. This shows that using SCF through Ultipor SQ40S without infusion of the buffy coat, the TRR was 1.4% and the PRR 11%. It is interesting to compare these values with those collected in the same clinical setting in previous periods, when different techniques were used to prepare leucocyte-poor red cells. In 1980, 1981 and 1982, when the 35 'more reactive' patients were transfused with leucocyte-poor red cells prepared by double centrifugation, the TRR of the whole group were 12.9%, 11.3% and 9.8%, respectively; in 1983 and 1984, when filtration through Imugard was used for the 35 'more reactive'. patients above, the TRR of the whole group dropped to 2.0% and 1.0%, respectively. The decrease of TRR was accompanied by a decrease of PRR. The use of SCF through Ultipor SQ40S without infusion of the buffy coat, therefore, gave values as good as those of the Imugard period. Whilst showing the same efficacy as one of the most effective available techniques,

Table 6.4 Comparison of the efficacy of the standard administration filter (170 μ) with that of Ultipor SQ40S in the Spin, Cool and Filter technique without infusion of the buffy coat (from Parravicini et al 1986).

Filters used	Pairs of PRC[1] units processed (No.)	Red cell recovery (%)	Residual leucocytes ($\times 10^6$)	Granulocytes (given as percentage of residual leucocytes)
Standard (170 μ)	15	85[2] (75–95)[3]	330 (85–1390)	15
Ultipor SQ40S (40 μ)	15	82 (77–96)	125 (51–287)	12

[1] Packed red cells 4–7 days old
[2] Median
[3] Range

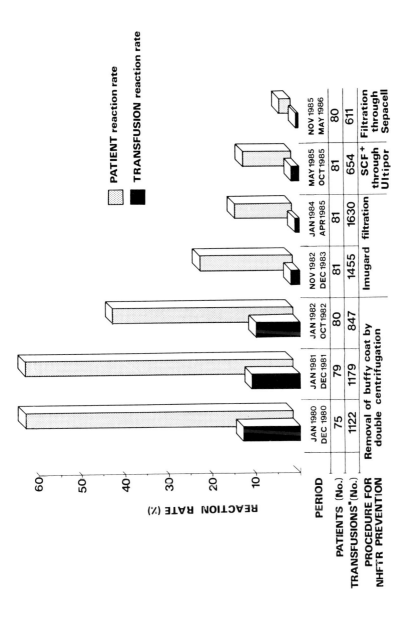

Fig. 6.1 Transfusion and patient reaction rates recorded in different years in a group of thalassaemic patients (from Sirchia et al 1987).

SCF through Ultipor SQ40S offered other advantages. As noted previously, the blood bag was not entered before transfusion and the cost of the procedure was low both in the transfusion centre and in the clinical setting. In the ward the work of the nurse was reduced: most patients aged 8 years or more were willing to cooperate in their treatment and became skilled in stopping the transfusion at the right moment: one nurse could manage up to 10 patients at a time. The major drawback of the method was the need to handle the bag carefully so as to avoid disruption of the buffy coat.

The goal is now to prepare a filter to be used at the bedside capable of retaining all contaminating leucocytes without special manoeuvres. Such a filter is in sight: recently Sepacell R-500 ®️ (Asahi, Japan) has been made commercially available. This is a filter which combines screening and adsorption, and allows leucocyte-free (or -very poor) red cells to be trans-fused at the bedside in a median time of 65 min/unit without needing to spin and cool the blood bags previously or to stop the transfusion to prevent infusion of the buffy coat. We evaluated Sepacell in the same clinical setting and with the same study design reported above for SCF through Ultipor SQ40S (Sirchia et al 1987). We obtained a TRR of 0.5% and a PRR of 3.7% (Fig. 1) which were not unexpected in view of the high purity of the filtered blood. By administering 2 PRC units per filter, no leucocytes were detectable in 17% of transfusions, 1 to 12×10^6 in 58% of transfusions and 13 to 100×10^6 leucocytes in the other 25%. Results of the in vitro evaluation of Sepacell are reported in detail in Table 6.5.

Unfortunately Sepacell is not yet the final answer, especially because of the poor red cell recovery; only if 2 blood units are administered through 1 filter did the red cell recovery become acceptable. Moreover the median infusion time of 65 min, with a range of 25–180, inhibits the use of Sepacell in the operating theatre. If red cells are suspended in saline or saline-adenine-glucose-mannitol (SAG-mannitol) solution, however, the infusion time is considerably reduced while allowing satisfactory leucocyte (and platelet) depletion and acceptable red cell recovery.

Table 6.5 In vitro effectiveness of Sepacell filtration of packed red cell units prepared from blood collected in CPDA-1 (CPDA-PRC) or from blood collected in CPD and resuspended in the SAG-Mannitol solution (SAGMAN-PRC) (from Sirchia et al 1987).

Type of red cell unit filtered	No. of PRC[1] units per filter	Red cell recovery (%)	Residual leucocytes ($\times 10^6$)	Residual platelets ($\times 10^9$)
CPDA-PRC	1	74.0[2] (68.2–80.6)[3]	0 (0–11)	1.3 (0.2–5.4)
(n = 60)	2	87.0 (83.0–92.0)	6.1 (0–100)	2.7 (0.6–9.7)
SAGMAN-PRC	1	83.0 (75.0–90.0)	2 (0–6)	1.7 (0.3–5.1)
(n = 40)	2	91.0 (85.0–100.0)	8 (0–22)	2.6 (0.7–6.7)

[1] Packed red cells 1–14 days old
[2] Median
[3] Range

SUMMARY

Leucocytes that contaminate all standard blood components can be the cause of important transfusion complications, including the production of antileucocyte antibodies (that in turn can determine nonhaemolytic febrile transfusion reactions, refractoriness to platelet transfusion and rejection of transplants), transmission of some viruses, immune depression, and graft-versus-host disease.

Methods for the preparation of leucocyte-poor red cells can be divided into those which, because they require more or less sophisticated manoeuvres, must be used in the transfusion centre, and those which can be used at the bedside. The first group of procedures includes 5 basic techniques (although many methodological variants of these techniques exist): differential centrifugation, sedimentation, cell washing, freezing and thawing, and filtration. Whereas differential centrifugation for the preparation of buffy coat-depleted red cells still has a role, the next three procedures have today only limited indications for the preparation of leucocyte-poor blood and are being replaced by filtration. The two most popular filters for this use are Imugard IG-500 (containing cotton wool) and Erypur (containing cellulose acetate). The former is also suitable for the preparation of leucocyte-free platelet concentrates, and both filters (especially Erypur) can produce leucocyte-free red cell units. This is expected to provide the means for preventing or delaying the production of antileucocyte antibodies in previously nonstimulated candidates for prolonged transfusion treatment. Methods for the production of leucocyte-depleted red cells at the bedside include 'Spin, Cool and Filter' through the filter for microaggregates Ultipor SQ40S and filtration of the unprocessed blood unit through Sepacell R-500. This latter filter allows the transfusion of leucocyte-free (or -very poor) red cells, but results are not reproducible since the infusion time of the blood is sometimes prolonged unacceptably. The red cell recovery, moreover, is low if 1 blood unit is administered through the filter and becomes acceptable only if 2 units are transfused through the same filter. The ideal filter, capable of producing leucocyte-free red cells at the bedside without the need of any skill or special manoeuvre at reasonable cost, is now in sight. If such a filter becomes available we should consider using it for every transfused patient in place of the usual blood administration filter of 170 μ. This policy, proposed a few years ago (Goldfinger and Lowe, 1981) but unrealistic at that time, might now become feasible and constitute a major step forward in transfusion therapy.

AKNOWLEDGEMENTS

The authors are grateful to the medical students F. Bertolini, F. Marangoni, and D. Prati for their enthusiastic participation in this work, to A. M. Green for help in preparing the manuscript and to D. Notari for secretarial assistance. Grant no 85.02377.44 of CNR, Rome.

Appendix: Comparison of the principal procedures for the preparation of leucocyte-depleted red cells for transfusion

Procedure	Reference (first author and year)	Residual leucocytes ($\times 10^6$)	Leucocyte removal (%)	Red cell recovery (%)	Comments
Removal of buffy coat	Prins (1980)	1100 ± 600	> 60%	nr	inexpensive buffy coat removed = 40–50 g
	Högman (1981)	1050 ± 450	69 ± 11	~ 90	
Inverted spin	Tenczar (1973)	550 ± 350	80.4 ± 13.6	76.0 ± 4.9	time-consuming
	Meryman (1980)	330 ± 310	88.4 ± 6.9	68.7 ± 5.6	
Upright spin (of diluted PRC)	Meryman (1980)	160 ± 60	90 ± 3.4	88.6 ± 3.5	time-consuming
Double sedimentation					open system, time-consuming
— Dextran	Chaplin (1959)	nr	97.5	>98	
	Sirchia (1980)	no detectable leucocytes in 25% of cases; 1–50 × 10⁶ in 72% of cases	nr	86 (85–87)	
— HES	Dorner (1975)	nr	95.5	~ 90	
Machine washing					open system, not cost-effective
— IBM	Wooten (1976)	nr	84.7	85.5	
	Bryant (1978)	nr	93.3	82.1	
	Lichtiger (1984)	nr	87.8 ± 6.8	87 ± 6.8	
	Uda (1984)	nr	93.8	87.8	
— Haemonetics	Wenz (1980a)	650 ± 280	68.4 ± 14	83.7	
Freezing and thawing					open system, not cost-effective
— high glycerol	Crowley (1974b)	320	91	94	
	Polesky (1977)	40.7 no detectable leucocytes in 79% of cases	> 98	nr	
— low glycerol	Crowley (1974b)	80	> 97	92	

Filtration in the transfusion centre

— Imugard	Sirchia (1982b)	no detectable leucocytes in 30% of cases; 1–50 × 10^6 in 70% of cases	nr	87 (86–88)	open system
	Feng (1984)	nr	~ 96	~ 90	
	Lichtiger (1984)	nr	94.1 ± 5.2	91.1 ± 8.7	
— Erypur	Diepenhorst (1975)	no detectable leucocytes in 66% of cases	> 98	96 ± 16	
	Elghouzzi (1981)	42.4	98 ± 2	92 ± 6.5	
	Sirchia (1982b)	no detectable leucocytes in 62% of cases; 1–50 × 10^6 in 38% of cases	nr	93 (91–94)	

Filtration at the bedside

— SF – Ultipor SQ40S	Wenz (1983)	600	83	94 ± 2	easy, inexpensive, closed system
— SF – Fenwal 4C2423	Wenz (1983)	600	83	88 ± 4	not suitable for fresh blood
— SF – Ultipor SQ40S	Parravicini (1984)	920 (150–1400)	71 (70–83)	90.3 (83–97)	
— SCF – Ultipor SQ40S	Parravicini (1984)	360 (110–1100)	84 (82–92)	92.7 (82–98)	PRC 4–9 days old
— SCF – Ultipor SQ40S (without infusion of buffy coat)	Parravicini (1984)	130 (20–300)	95 (92–97)	80.1 (70–90)	
— Sepacell R-500	Sirchia (1987)	no detectable leucocytes in 53% of cases; 1–11 × 10^6 in 47% of cases	nr	74.0 (68.2–80.6)	suitable for preparation of leucocyte-free (or -very poor) red cells even using fresh blood; infusion time variable from filter to filter

nr = not reported; PRC = packed red cells; SF = Spin and Filter; SCF = Spin, Cool and Filter.

REFERENCES

Adler S P, Baggett J, McVoy M 1985 Transfusion-associated cytomegalovirus infections in seropositive cardiac surgery patients. Lancet 2: 743–746

Amer K A, Pepper D S, Urbaniak S J 1980 Lymphocyte, granulocyte and platelet contamination of blood frozen by the low-glycerol liquid nitrogen technique. British Journal of Haematology 44: 253–261

Andreu G, Lam Y Y, Devers L, Rio B 1986 Routine use of Imugard filters for preparation of leucocyte depleted random platelet concentrates. 21st Congress of the International Society of Haematology – 19th Congress of the International Society of Blood Transfusion, Sydney, 1986. Book of Abstracts, p 498

Barton J C 1981 Nonhemolytic, noninfectious transfusion reactions. Seminars in Hematology 18: 95–121

Blumberg N, Agarwal M M, Chuang C 1985 Relation between recurrence of cancer of the colon and blood transfusion. British Medical Journal 290: 1037–1039

Bollinger R R, Sanfilippo F, Spees E K, Vaughn W K, Hawthorne R 1982 Renal transplantation in highly sensitized patients. Transplantation Proceedings 14: 46–48

Brand A 1985 Personal communication

Brittingham T E, Chaplin H jr 1957 Febrile transfusion reactions caused by sensitivity to donor leukocytes and platelets. Journal of the American Medical Association 165: 819–825

Bryant L R, Holland L, Corkern S 1978 Optimal leukocyte removal from refrigerated blood with the IBM 2991 Blood Cell Processor. Transfusion 18: 469–471

Burrows L, Tartter P 1982 Effect of blood transfusions on colonic malignancy recurrence rate. Lancet 2:662

Chaplin H jr 1982 The proper use of previously frozen red blood cells for transfusion. Blood 59: 1118–1120

Chaplin H jr, Brittingham T E, Cassel M 1959 Methods for preparation of suspensions of buffy coat-poor red blood cells for transfusion. Including a report of 50 transfusions of suspensions of buffy coat-poor red blood cells prepared by a dextran sedimentation method. American Journal of Clinical Pathology 31: 373–383

Crowley J P, Valeri C R 1974a The purification of red cells for transfusion by freeze preservation and washing. II. The residual leukocytes, platelets, and plasma in washed, freeze-preserved red cells. Transfusion 14: 196–202

Crowley J P, Valeri C R 1974b The purification of red cells for transfusion by freeze-preservation and washing. III. Leukocyte removal and red cell recovery after red cell freeze-preservation by the high or low glycerol concentration method. Transfusion 14: 590–594

Cullen D J, Ferrara L 1974 Comparative evaluation of blood filters: a study in vitro. Anesthesiology 41: 568–575

Décary F, Ferner P, Giavedoni L, et al 1984 An investigation of nonhemolytic transfusion reactions. Vox Sanguinis 46: 277–285

De Martino M, Rossi M E, Muccioli A T, Vullo C, Vierucci A 1985 Altered T cell subsets and function in polytransfused beta-thalassemia patients: correlation with sex and age at first transfusion. Vox Sanguinis 48: 296–304

De Rie M A, Plas-van Dalen C M van der, Engelfriet C P, Borne A E G Kr von dem 1985 The serology of febrile transfusion reactions. Vox Sanguinis 49: 126–134

Diepenhorst P, Engelfriet C P 1975 Removal of leukocytes from whole blood and erythrocyte suspensions by filtration through cotton wool. V. Results after transfusion of 1820 units of filtered erythrocytes. Vox Sanguinis 29: 15–21

Diepenhorst P, Sprokholt R, Prins H K 1972 Removal of leukocytes from whole blood and erythrocyte suspensions by filtration through cotton wool. I. Filtration technique. Vox Sanguinis 23: 308–320

Dorner I, Moore J A, Collins J A, Sherman L A, Chaplin H jr 1975 Efficacy of leucocyte-poor red blood cell suspensions prepared by sedimentation in hydroxyethyl starch. Transfusion 15: 439–448

Duquesnoy R J, Filip D J, Rodey G E, Rimm A A, Aster R H 1977 Successful transfusion of platelets 'mismatched' for HLA antigens to alloimmunized thrombocytopenic patients. American Journal of Hematology 2: 219–226

Eernisse J G, Brand A 1981 Prevention of platelet refractoriness due to HLA antibodies by administration of leukocyte-poor blood components. Experimental Hematology 9: 77–83

Elghouzzi M H, Vedrenne J B, Jullien A M, Delcey D, Nadal M, Habibi B 1981 Etude technique immunologique et clinique des performances de filtration du sang à l'aide de l'appareil Erypur. Revue Française de Transfusion et Immunohématologie 24: 579–595

Engelfriet C P, Diepenhorst P, Giessen M von der, Riesz E von 1975 Removal of leukocytes from whole blood and erythrocyte suspensions by filtration through cotton wool. IV. Immunization studies in rabbits. Vox Sanguinis 28: 81–89

Feng C S, de Jongh D S, Bouchette D, Wallace M E, Kao Y S 1984 Evaluation of cotton-wool filters for preparing leukocyte-poor blood. Laboratory Medicine 15: 47–49

Ford J M, Lucey J J, Cullen M H, Tobias J S, Lister T A·1976 Fatal graft-versus-host disease following transfusion of granulocytes from normal donors. Lancet 2: 1167–1169

Foster R S jr, Costanza M C, Foster J C, Wanner M C, Foster C B 1985 Adverse relationship between blood transfusions and survival after colectomy for colon cancer. Cancer 55: 1195–1201

Gascòn P, Zoumbos N C, Young N S 1984 Immunologic abnormalities in patients receiving multiple blood transfusions. Annals of Internal Medicine 100: 173–177

Goldfinger D, Lowe C 1981 Prevention of adverse reactions to blood transfusion by the administration of saline-washed red blood cells. Transfusion 21: 277–280

Grady R W, Akbar A N, Giardina P J, Hilgartner M W, de Sousa M 1985 Disproportionate lymphoid cell subsets in thalassaemia major: the relative contributions of transfusion and splenectomy. British Journal of Haematology 59: 713–724

Greenwalt T J, Gajewski M, McKenna J L 1962 A new method for preparing buffy coat-poor blood. Transfusion 2: 221–229

Hathaway W E, Fulginiti V A, Pierce C W et al 1967 Graft-versus-host reaction following a single blood transfusion. Journal of the American Medical Association 201: 1015–1020

Herzig R H, Herzig G P, Bull M I et al 1975 Correction of poor platelet transfusion responses with leukocyte-poor HL-A-matched platelet concentrates. Blood 46: 743–750

Hewson J W, Dickeson L, Lovric V A 1986 Efficiency of cotton wool filtration in removing leukocytes and preserving platelet yield and function from concentrates. 21st Congress of the International Society of Haematology – 19th Congress of the International Society of Blood Transfusion, Sydney, 1986. Book of Abstracts, p 497

Högman C F, Johansson A 1981 A simple method for the preparation of microaggregate-poor whole blood. Vox Sanguinis 40: 286–288

Högman C F 1986 Personal communication

Howard J E, Perkins H A 1978 The natural history of alloimmunization to platelets. Transfusion 18: 496–503

Huang S T, Helton M R, Floyd D M, McGowan E I 1985 The preparation of leukocyte-poor red cells from AS-1 blood by modified microaggregate filtration technique. 38th Annual Meeting, American Association of Blood Banks. Transfusion 25:454 (Abstract S36)

Hughes A S B, Brozović B 1982 Leucocyte depleted blood: an appraisal of available techniques. British Journal of Haematology 50: 381–386

Hurley M J, Miller E, de Jongh D S, Litwin M S 1978 Filtration characteristics of the Dual-Mode (Johnson and Johnson) micropore blood transfusion filter. Transfusion 18: 582–587

Hyman N H, Foster R S jr, De Meules J E, Costanza M C 1985 Blood transfusions and survival after lung cancer resection. The American Journal of Surgery 149: 502–507

Kaplan J, Sarnaik S, Gitlin J, Lusher J 1984 Diminished helper/suppressor lymphocyte ratios and natural killer activity in recipients of repeated blood transfusions. Blood 64: 308–310

Kikugawa K, Minoshima K 1978 Filter columns for preparation of leukocyte-poor blood for transfusion. Vox Sanguinis 34: 281–290

Kissmeyer-Nielsen F, Olsen S, Petersen Posborg V, Fjeldborg O 1966 Hyperacute rejection of kidney allografts associated with pre-existing humoral antibodies against donor cells. Lancet 2: 662–665

Koerner K, Kubanek B 1987 Comparison of three different methods used in the preparation of leukocyte-poor platelet concentrates. Vox Sanguinis 53: 26–30

Koerner K, Stampe D 1982 Preparation of leucocyte- and platelet-poor red cell concentrates. Blut 44: 305–308

Kurtz S R, Valeri D A, Melaragno A J et al 1981 Leukocyte-poor red blood cells prepared by the addition and removal of glycerol from red blood cell concentrates stored at 4°C. Transfusion 21: 435–442

Leng B, Chong C, Lovric V A, Wisdom L, Spencer S, Carmen R A 1984 Simple and economical preparation of leukocyte poor red cells. 37th Annual Meeting, American Association of Blood Banks. Transfusion 24:419 (Abstract S17)

Lichtiger B, del Valle L, Armintor M, Trujillo J M 1984 Use of Imugard IG500 filters for preparation of leukocyte-poor blood for cancer patients. Vox Sanguinis 46: 136–141

Liedén G, Hildén J-O 1982 Febrile transfusion reactions reduced by use of buffy-coat-poor erythrocyte concentrates. Vox Sanguinis 43: 263–265

Lovric V A, Schuller M, Raftos J, Wisdom L 1981 Filtered microaggregate-free erythrocyte concentrates with 35-day shelf life. Vox Sanguinis 41: 6–10

Lowe G D 1981 Filtration in intravenous therapy. IV. Blood filters. British Journal of Intravenous Therapy 2: 47–54

Masse M, Naegelen C, Coffe C, Blanchard R, Peters A 1986 Comparative study of the different techniques of leukocyte-free platelet concentrates. 21st Congress of the International Society of Haematology – 19th Congress of the International Society of Blood Transfusion, Sydney, 1986. Book of Abstracts, p 498

McNamara J J, Boatright D, Burran E L, Molot M D, Summers E, Stremple J F 1971 Changes in some physical properties of stored blood. Annals of Surgery 174: 58–60

Menitove J E, McElligott M C, Aster R H 1982 Febrile transfusion reaction: what blood component should be given next? Vox Sanguinis 42: 318–321

Meryman H T, Bross J, Lebovitz R 1980 The preparation of leukocyte-poor red blood cells: a comparative study. Transfusion 20: 285–292

Meryman H T, Hornblower M 1986 The preparation of red cells depleted of leukocytes. Review and evaluation. Transfusion 26: 101–106

Mijović V, Brozović B, Hughes A S B, Davies T D 1983 Leukocyte-depleted blood. A comparison of filtration techniques. Transfusion 23: 30–32

Milner G R, Fagence R, Darnborough J 1982 Temperature dependence of leukocyte depletion of blood with an automatic blood cell processor. Transfusion 22: 48–50

Minchinton R M, Waters A H, Baker L R I, Cattell W R 1980 Platelet, granulocyte, and HLA antibodies in renal dialysis patients transfused with frozen blood. British Medical Journal 281: 113–114

Munn C G, Markenson A L, Kapadia A, deSousa M 1981 Impaired T-cell mitogen responses in some patients with thalassaemia intermedia. Thymus 3: 119–128

Murphy M F, Metcalfe P, Thomas H et al 1986 Use of leucocyte-poor blood components and HLA-matched-platelet donors to prevent HLA alloimmunization. British Journal of Haematology 62: 529–534

Myllylä G, Ruutu T, Oksanen L, Rasi V, Kekomäki R 1986 Preparation and properties of leukocyte-free platelet concentrates. 21st Congress of the International Society of Haematology – 19th Congress of the International Society of Blood Transfusion, Sydney, 1986. Book of Abstracts, p 498

Neri A, Brugiatelli M, Iacopino P, Callea V, Ronco F 1984 Natural killer cell activity and T subpopulations in thalassemia major. Acta Haematologica 71: 263–269

Opelz G 1985 Effect of HLA matching, blood transfusions and presensitization in Cyclosporine-treated kidney transplant recipients. Transplantation Proceedings 17: 2179–2183

Opelz G, Sengar D P S, Mickey M R, Terasaki P I 1973 Effect of blood transfusions on subsequent kidney transplants. Transplantation Proceedings 5: 253–259

Parravicini A, Morelati F, Rebulla P, Bertolini F, Sirchia G 1983 Emocomponenti poveri e privi di leucociti. Centro Trasfusionale Ospedale Maggiore Policlinico di Milano Editore, Milano

Parravicini A, Rebulla P, Apuzzo J, Wenz B, Sirchia G 1984 The preparation of leukocyte-poor red cells for transfusion by a simple cost-effective technique. Transfusion 24: 508–509

Parravicini A, Rebulla P, Bertolini F et al 1987 Clinical evaluation of the Spin, Cool and Filter technique for the preparation of leukocyte-poor red blood cells at the bedside. In: Sirchia G, Zanella A (eds) Thalassemia today (Proceedings of the Second Mediterranean

Meeting on Thalassemia, Milano, 1985), Centro Transfusionale Ospedale Maggiore Policlinico di Milano Editore, Milano, p 45–51

Payne R 1957 The association of febrile transfusion reactions with leuko-agglutinins. Vox Sanguinis 2: 233–241

Perkins H A 1977 HLA antigens and blood transfusion: effect on renal transplants. Transplantation Proceedings 9 (suppl 1): 229–232

Perkins H A, Payne R, Ferguson J, Wood M 1966 Nonhemolityc febrile transfusion reactions. Quantitative effects of blood components with emphasis on isoantigenic incompatibility of leukocytes. Vox Sanguinis 11: 578–600

Persijn G G, Cohen B, Lansbergen Q, van Rood J J 1979 Retrospective and prospective studies on the effect of blood transfusions in renal transplantation in the Netherlands. Transplantation 28: 396–401

Polesky H F 1977 Leukocyte-poor blood, a study in the evolution of component therapy. In: A seminar on blood components: e unum pluribus. American Association of Blood Banks, Washington DC, p 53–74

Polesky H F, McCullough J, Helgeson M A, Nelson C 1973 Evaluation of methods for the preparation of HL-A antigen-poor blood. Transfusion 13: 383–387

Prins H K, de Bruijn J C G H, Henrichs H P J, Loos J A 1980 Prevention of microaggregate formation by removal of 'buffy-coats'. In: Symposium on Microfiltration of Blood and Pulmonary Function. Vox Sanguinis 39: 48–51

Prins H K, Henrichs H P J, Conemans J M H, Leurink H J, Krijnen H W 1978 Preparation of leukocyte-poor red cell suspensions from 'buffy-coat'-free red cell concentrates by simplified cotton wool filtration. 17th Congress of the International Society of Hematology – 15th Congress of the International Society of Blood Transfusion, Paris, 1978. Abstract Volume I, p 147

Rebulla P, Sirchia G 1985 (unpublished data)

Reesink H W, Veldman H, Henrichs H J, Prins H K, Loos J A 1982 Removal of leukocytes from blood by fibre filtration. A comparison study on the performance of two commercially available filters. Vox Sanguinis 42: 281–288

Reynolds L O, Simon T L 1980 Size distribution measurements of microaggregates in stored blood. Transfusion 20: 669–678

Rinaldo C R jr, Black P H, Hirsh M S 1977 Interaction of cytomegalovirus with leucocytes from patients with mononucleosis due to cytomegalovirus. Journal of Infectious Diseases 136: 667–678

Robinson E A E 1984 Single donor granulocytes and platelets. Clinics in Haematology 13: 185–216

Rock G, Baxter A, Gray E 1984 Leukocyte-depleted blood: a comparison of available preparations. Canadian Medical Association Journal 130: 1566–1568

Schiffer C A, Lichtenfeld J L, Wiernik P H, Mardiney M R, Joseph J M 1976 Antibody response in patients with acute nonlymphocytic leukemia. Cancer 37: 2177–2182

Schiffer C A, Aisner J, Wiernik P H 1978 Frozen autologous platelet transfusion for patients with leukemia. New England Journal of Medicine 299: 7–12

Schiffer C A, Dutcher J P, Aisner J, Hogge D, Wiernik P H, Reilly J P 1983 A randomized trial of leukocyte-depleted platelet transfusion to modify alloimmunization in patients with leukemia. Blood 62: 815–820

Schmidt P J (Ed) 1984 Standards for blood banks and transfusion services. XI edition. American Association of Blood Banks, Arlington, VA, p 10

Schned A R, Silver H 1981 The use of microaggregate filtration in the prevention of febrile transfusion reactions. Transfusion 21: 675–681

Schneider W, Stützle G 1979 Neues Verfahren zur Herstellung von leukozyten-thrombozytenarmen Erythrozytensedimenten. Medizinische Welt (Stuttgart) 30: 1597–1601

Schrier R D, Nelson J A, Oldstone M B A 1985 Detection of human Cytomegalovirus in peripheral blood lymphocytes in a natural infection. Science 230: 1048–1051

Scornik J C, Ireland J E, Howard R J, Fennell R S, Pfaff W W 1984 Role of regular and leukocyte-free blood transfusions in the generation of broad sensitization. Transplantation 38: 594–598

Shimizu T, Ishikawa Y, Tsurumi H et al 1986 Method for processing leukocyte- and platelet- poor red cells in closed bags. Vox Sanguinis 50: 203–207

Sintnicolaas K 1986 Preparation of leukocyte-free platelets by cotton-wool filtration: in vitro and in vivo evaluation. 21st Congress of the International Society of Haematology – 19th Congress of the International Society of Blood Transfusion, Sydney, 1986. Book of Abstracts, p 497

Sirchia G, Parravicini A, Rebulla P, Fattori L, Milani S 1980 Evaluation of three procedures for the preparation of leukocyte-poor and leukocyte-free red blood cells for transfusion. Vox Sanguinis 38: 197–204

Sirchia G, Mercuriali F, Pizzi C, Rosso di San Secondo V E M, Borzini P, Aniasi A 1982a Blood transfusion and kidney transplantation: effect of small doses of blood on kidney graft function and survival. Transplantation Proceedings 14: 263–271

Sirchia G, Parravicini A, Rebulla P, Greppi N, Scalamogna M, Morelati F 1982b Effectiveness of red blood cells filtered through cotton wool to prevent antileukocyte antibody production in multitransfused patients. Vox Sanguinis 42: 190–197

Sirchia G, Parravicini A, Rebulla P, Bertolini F, Morelati F, Marconi M 1983 Preparation of leukocyte-free platelets for transfusion by filtration through cotton wool. Vox Sanguinis 44: 115–120

Sirchia G, Rebulla P, Mascaretti L et al 1986 The clinical importance of leukocyte depletion in regular erythrocyte transfusions. Vox Sanguinis 51 (Suppl. 1): 2–8

Sirchia G, Rebulla P, Parravicini A, Carnelli V, Gianotti G A, Bertolini F 1987 Leukocyte depletion of red cell units at the bedside by transfusion through a new filter. Transfusion (in press)

Sniecinski I, O'Donnell M 1986 White cell depletion of blood products by cotton-wool filtration. An economical method for decreasing alloimmunization in multiply transfused patients. 21st Congress of the International Society of Haematology – 19th Congress of the International Society of Blood Transfusion, Sydney, 1986. Book of Abstracts, p 574

Sniecinski I, St Jean J, Nowicki B 1986 Preparation of leukocyte-poor platelet concentrates. Journal of Plasma Therapy and Transfusion Technology (in press)

Solis R T, Gibbs M B 1972 Filtration of the microaggregates in stored blood. Transfusion 12: 245–250

Solis R T, Goldfinger D, Gibbs M B, Zeller J A 1974 Physical characteristics of microaggregates in stored blood. Transfusion 14: 538–550

Swank R L 1961 Alteration of blood on storage: measurement of adhesiveness of 'aging' platelets and leukocytes and their removal by filtration. New England Journal of Medicine 265: 728–733

Tenczar F J 1973 Comparison of inverted centrifugation, saline washing, and dextran sedimentation in the preparation of leukocyte-poor red cells. Transfusion 13: 183–188

Treleaven J G, Patterson K G, Blagdon J 1982 Comparative study of the Fenwal and Pall microaggregate filters used for the production of leukocyte-poor blood. Journal of Clinical Pathology 35: 681–683

Uda M, Naito S, Yamamoto K, Ishii A, Nishizaki T 1984 Optimal protocol for preparation of leukocyte-poor red cells with a blood cell processor. Transfusion 24: 120–123

Vakkila J, Myllylä G 1986 Characterization of leukocyte-free red cell and platelet concentrates. 1st European Symposium on Quality in Blood Transfusion, Strasbourg, 1986. Abstract Volume, p 13

Valeri C R, Valeri D A, Anastasi J, Vecchione J J, Dennis R C, Emerson C P 1981 Freezing in the primary polyvinylchloride plastic collection bag: a new system for preparing and freezing nonrejuvenated and rejuvenated red blood cells. Transfusion 21: 138–149

Verdonck L F, Middeldorp J M, Kreeft H A G, Hauw The T, Hekker A, de Gast G C 1985 Primary cytomegalovirus infection and its prevention after autologous bone marrow transplantation. Transplantation 39: 455–457

Vos J J E, Schoen C, Prins H K, Borne A E G Kr von dem, Huisman J G 1987 Monitoring of platelet contamination in filtered red blood cell concentrates. Vox Sanguinis 53: 23–25

Wenz B 1983 Microaggregate blood filtration and the febrile transfusion reaction. A comparative study. Transfusion 23: 95–98

Wenz B 1986 Leukocyte-poor blood. CRC Clinical Laboratory Sciences 24: 1–20

Wenz B, Apuzzo J 1987 Leukocyte poor blood. Current perspectives and the description of a new prototype-hybrid filter. In: Sirchia G, Zanella A (eds) Thalassemia today:

(Proceedings of the 2nd Mediterranean Meeting on Thalassemia, Milano 1985). Centro Trasfusionale Ospedale Maggiore Policlinico di Milano Editore, Milano, p 41–44

Wenz B, Apuzzo J H, Ahuja K K 1980a The preparation of leukocyte-poor red cells from liquid stored blood: an evaluation of the Haemonetics ® 102 cell washing system. Transfusion 20: 306–310

Wenz B, Gurtlinger K F, O'Toole A M, Dugan E P 1980b Preparation of granulocyte-poor red blood cells by microaggregate filtration. A simplified method to minimize febrile transfusion reactions. Vox Sanguinis 39: 282–287

Wooten M J 1976 Use and analysis of saline washed red blood cells. Transfusion 16: 464–468

Yankee R A, Grumet F C, Rogentine G N 1969 Platelet transfusion therapy. The selection of compatible platelet donors for refractory patients by lymphocyte HL-A typing. New England Journal of Medicine 281: 1208–1212

Screening for anti-HTLV-III: experience in blood centres in the United States and the United Kingdom

INTRODUCTION

Although a number of methodologies have been devised to detect antibody to the human T-lymphotropic virus type III (anti-HTLV-III), this review will focus on the development, licensure in the United States (USA), and experience with enzyme-linked immunosorbent assays (ELISA) intended to detect individuals exposed to the aetiologic agent of acquired immunodeficiency syndrome (AIDS). Other methods to detect anti-HTLV-III, namely Western blot and indirect immunofluorescence (IFA), will only be mentioned in the context of confirmatory testing of samples giving reactive results in the ELISA screening test. A chronological narrative of the development and use of the ELISA test in USA blood centres will be supplemented by a comparison to the experience in the UK. Recent concensus recommendations have proposed adopting the term human immunodeficiency virus (HIV) (Coffin et al 1986) to refer to both HTLV-III and lymphadenopathy-associated virus (LAV); however, in the context of this review we feel it necessary to retain the original terminology for purposes of clarity. The authors hope that the rapid spread of the AIDS epidemic and the equally rapid response of the scientific community which resulted in the isolation of LAV and the subsequent development of the ELISA test for anti-HTLV-III, will not date the information in this article before it reaches the reader.

A June 1981 report (CDC 1981) of biopsy-confirmed *Pneumocystis carinii* pneumonia in five young homosexually active men from Los Angeles, California was the first to call attention to the syndrome now known as AIDS.

The occurrence of *P. carinii* pneumonia in three haemophilia A patients during 1982 (CDC 1982) suggested that an infectious agent in Factor VIII might be responsible for the immune dysfunction seen in these patients. The similarity of the epidemiology of AIDS to hepatitis B further strengthened the hypothesis that AIDS was caused by an infectious agent. With the report of AIDS in a recipient of single donor blood and blood components (Ammann et al 1983) the stage was set for a meeting held in Atlanta,

110

Georgia on 4 January 1983, jointly sponsored by the Centers for Disease Control (CDC), the Food and Drug Administration (FDA), and the National Institutes of Health (NIH), which considered the possibility that AIDS was being transmitted by blood and blood products and concluded that transfusion-transmitted AIDS represented a real and imminent danger.

In an attempt to minimize the risk of transfusion-transmitted AIDS, USA blood and plasma facilities implemented guidelines for donor self-deferral in March 1983 (CDC 1983a) which specified that members of groups at increased risk for AIDS should refrain from donating blood or plasma.

In May 1983 three papers appeared in *Science* implicating human retroviruses as the possible cause of AIDS. One reported the isolation of human T-cell leukemia virus (HTLV-I) from the peripheral blood T-lymphocytes from several patients with AIDS (Gallo et al 1983). Antibodies to HTLV-I were found by IFA at much higher frequencies in patients with AIDS or the lymphadenopathy syndrome than in controls (Essex et al 1983). More importantly, a related but distinct retrovirus, the lymphadenopathy-associated virus (LAV), was isolated from cells from a lymph node of a patient with the lymphadenopathy syndrome (Barré-Sinoussi et al 1983).

The relatively low prevalence (circa 25%) of HTLV-I antibodies in AIDS patients led to speculation that a related retrovirus might be the responsible aetiologic agent of AIDS. In fact, LAV was that related virus, but the French investigators who discovered LAV failed to find a cell line in which the virus would replicate continuously and reach high titres. Hence, they were unable to produce antibody tests to do the necessary seroepidemiologic studies to establish the association of LAV with AIDS. This sine qua non was provided by USA scientists at NIH in the form of the H9 cell line (Popovic et al 1984) which enabled these investigators to obtain large volumes of high-titred retrovirus isolates, collectively termed HTLV-III, which originated from patients with AIDS or the lymphadenopathy syndrome. They were thus able to characterize the viruses biochemically, biophysically and immunologically. They further obtained 48 independent isolates of similar retroviruses from patients with AIDS and members of groups at risk for AIDS (Gallo et al 1984). Moreover, an ELISA test was described to detect antibodies to HTLV-III which showed high prevalences of infection in patients with AIDS or the lymphadenopathy syndrome and asymptomatic members of groups at risk for AIDS, whereas control populations were infected at low prevalence (Sarngadharan et al 1984). These studies unequivocally established the aetiologic role of HTLV-III in AIDS and provided the necessary reagents to make the screening of blood and plasma donors a reality.

DEVELOPMENT OF LICENSED SCREENING TESTS IN THE USA

In a remarkably rapid transfer of technology the USA government granted licenses to five USA pharmaceutical manufacturers giving them access to

HTLV-III and the H9 cell line (Culliton 1984). In alphabetical order, the companies are Abbott Laboratories, DuPont, ElectroNucleonics, Litton Bionetics (now Organon Teknika), and Travenol Genentech Diagnostics (now Clinical Assays). Their task was to bring to the marketplace sensitive, specific, reproducible ELISA antibody tests to screen blood and plasma donors for evidence of HTLV-III infection. The perceived public demands for ensuring the safety of the blood supply, bureaucratic rhetoric, and the spirit of competition provided the impetus to accomplish this within a brief span of time. Because of what was known about retrovirus biology at the time, an antibody test was deemed sufficient to detect individuals likely to transmit HTLV-III infection. The underlying assumptions were that all persons exposed to HTLV-III would rapidly become antibody positive and would carry intergrated HTLV-III DNA sequences in their lymphocytes indefinitely, thus making these persons potentially infectious.

Before conducting clinical trials, the manufacturers were required to show that their HTLV-III antigen preparation and other kit components, e.g. positive controls, were non-infectious. Furthermore, the kits had to perform satisfactorily on FDA proficiency panels. In addition, each manufacturer was required to test approximately 3000 plasma samples from a pool of 15 368 supplied to the FDA by blood collection facilities in different geographic regions of the USA during October 1984 (Petricianni et al 1985). This meant that the five companies tested different donor samples which precluded a direct comparison of their results. Of this donor cohort, 236 samples were reported to be repeatedly reactive (1.57%). Because sample volumes were limited, further testing by Western blot or IFA could not be done on most samples.

Clinical trials commenced in the fall of 1984. Arbitrary definitions of test sensitivity and specificity were established by the FDA at the time since there were no independent means to reliably identify infected and uninfected persons. It was assumed that all patients diagnosed with AIDS should have antibody to HTLV-III, whereas healthy individuals should not be infected. Thus, sensitivity was defined as the percentage of diagnosed AIDS patients who were positive by a given test, and specificity was the percentage of healthy individuals who were negative by a given test. Though the validity of these assumptions was questioned at the outset, they ultimately proved to be useful operational definitions.

Manufacturers engaged hospitals and clinics caring for AIDS patients as clinical sites for establishing sensitivity. Blood or plasma collection facilities conducted clinical trials to provide specificity data. Each manufacturer recruited its own clinical sites with the result that different sample collections were tested by each manufacturer, again precluding direct comparisons of the manufacturers' data. All used Western blot as a supplemental test for HTLV-III antibody detection to 'confirm' repeatedly reactive samples in the ELISA test; however, final sensitivity and specificity figures were calculated without reference to Western blot results.

Each of the five manufacturers' tests is based on the same design, that is, a sandwich assay. In brief, HTLV-III in culture supernatants from infected H9 cells is concentrated and then partially purified by density gradient centrifugation. The virus preparation is then detergent-disrupted and sonicated to inactivate infectious virus and to expose the internal antigens of the virus. The partially purified, disrupted, inactivated antigen is then adsorbed onto a solid phase consisting of a microtitre plate or bead. The antigen-coated solid phase is incubated with a dilution of the serum or plasma to be tested for anti-HTLV-III; a specified number of controls is included with each assay. If antibodies to HTLV-III are present, they will bind to the HTLV-III antigens present on the solid phase. After aspiration of unbound material and washing of the solid phase, goat anti-human IgG (heavy and light chain specific) conjugated with horseradish peroxidase is added. If antigen-antibody complexes are present on the solid phase, the conjugate will bind to them during this incubation step. Following aspiration of the unbound conjugate and washing of the solid phase, a substrate, usually ortho-phenylene diamine, is added. With further incubation, colour develops in proportion to the amount of anti-HTLV-III bound to the solid phase. Acid is then added to stop the enzyme-substrate reaction, whereupon samples and controls are read spectrophotometrically to determine the test cutoff and identify reactive samples.

Each of these five manufacturers tested approximately 100 to 250 specimens from AIDS patients to establish sensitivity; specificity claims were developed from test data on 3500 to over 16 000 blood or plasma donors. The first manufacturer was licensed by the FDA on 2 March 1985 and selected blood collection facilities were screening donors by 4 March. Within the next 30 days two additional tests were licensed. The remaining two test kits were licensed in October 1985.

Since 1 January 1986 test kits from Genetic Systems and Ortho Diagnostics have been licensed by FDA. The latter is derived from HTLV-III and the H9 cell line, whereas the former uses LAV and a cell line designated CEM to produce viral antigen. The most recent sensitivity and specificity claims of all currently licensed HTLV-III/LAV test kits are

Table 7.1 Sensitivity and specificity of licensed HTLV-III/LAV ELISA test kits in the United States.

Manufacturer	% Sensitivity	% Specificity
Abbott	98.3	99.8
Dupont	99.3	99.7
ElectroNucleonics	99.6	99.2
Genetic Systems	100.0	99.8
Litton Bionetics*	98.9	99.6
Ortho	99.3	99.7
Travenol Genentech**	100.00	99.2

* Now Organon Teknika
** Now Clinical Assays. The test is not commercially available.

found in Table 7.1. Most of this data derives from the clinical trials conducted by each manufacturer. All kits showed excellent sensitivity, ranging from 98.3% to 100%, while retaining high specificity in the range of 99.2% to 99.8%.

IMPLEMENTATION OF SCREENING IN THE USA

Blood and plasma donor screening was rapidly implemented in the USA; by the summer of 1985 all collections were being screened for evidence of HTLV-III infection. The following format for interdicting donations reactive for anti-HTLV-III has been followed by USA collection facilities: samples found reactive in an initial screen are tested in duplicate in a subsequent run. If two of three or three of three test results are reactive, the sample is said to be repeatedly reactive, and the donation is discarded. The donor is placed on a deferral list, and subsequent donations, even if they are non-reactive by ELISA, are discarded. Samples from ELISA-reactive donors are further tested by Western blot, the de facto confirmatory assay; those who are reactive are notified of their test results. In some regions donors who are non-reactive by Western blot are also told of their reactive ELISA test results. Policy makers are currently divided on the issue of notifying ELISA-reactive, Western blot non-reactive donors, but as of July 1986 voluntary blood collection facilities providing approximately two-thirds of the blood supply were not notifying such donors. All ELISA-reactive paid plasma donors have been informed of their results since the outset of screening by the commercial plasmapheresis industry.

An FDA study, begun soon after the first ELISA kits were licensed, monitored test data on approximately 2.5 million blood donations and a similar number of plasma donations (Kuritsky et al 1986). Of the blood donations 1.01% were initially reactive and 0.34% were repeatedly reactive. Similar rates were seen between donations from men and women. For source plasma donations the repeat reactive rate was 0.15%. Screening results were seen to vary geographically, with time, and by kit manufacturer for both blood and plasma collections. For short time periods the repeat reactive rate obtained with one manufacturer's assay was five- to tenfold greater than the yearly average. This increase in repeat reactive samples did not, however, correlate with an increase in confirmed Western blot reactivity.

Results from two reports from the American Red Cross regional blood centres (Schorr et al 1985, Sandler 1986) which exclusively used Abbott kits are summarized in Table 7.2. 40–50% of the repeatedly reactive samples having low sample to cutoff ratios (< 2) by ELISA were non-reactive with different kit lots. The small but significant increase in repeatedly reactive samples from 0.17% in May 1985 to 0.33% by February 1986 was probably due to an increase in false positives, because the percentage of Western blot positive donors declined slightly during this period.

Table 7.2 HTLV-III antibody test results from American Red Cross regional blood centres.

Donations Tested	Donations Initially Reactive	Donations Repeatedly Reactive	Donors Western Blot Positive
1 027 786	10 385 (1.01%)	1 723 (0.17%)	333[1] (0.032%)
5 500 000[2]	65 000 (1.18%)	18 000 (0.33%)	1675 (0.030%)

[1] Based on Western blot testing of 1455 of the 1723 repeatedly reactive donors
[2] This number includes the first 1 027 786 donations tested and represents results to February 1986

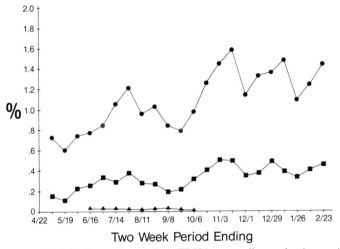

Fig. 7.1 % ELISA initially reactive (circles), ELISA repeatedly reactive (squares) and Western blot reactive (triangles) blood donations tested for antibody to HTLV-III. Data on 1 568 909 donations tested with Abbott kits from 22 April 1985 to 23 February 1986 were provided by 26 blood centres belonging to the Council of Community Blood Centers. (Reproduced with permission of the Council of Community Blood Centers.)

The variations with time in initially reactive, repeatedly reactive, and Western blot positive donor samples can be seen in Figure 7.1. ELISA test data on 1 568 909 donations were supplied by 26 regional blood centres belonging to the Council of Community Blood Centers. Small but significant swings in both initial- and repeat-reactive rates can be seen, especially in July 1985 and November-December 1985. Not shown in Figure 7.1 is an apparent downward trend in both initially and repeatedly reactive samples in March (1.01% and 0.28%, respectively) and April (0.57% and 0.14%, respectively) of 1986. Significantly the % of Western blot positive samples remained constant during a 16 week period from 16 June 1985 to 6 October 1985 when ELISA test reactivity rose and then fell, suggesting that the increase in test reactivity was due to false positive test results. Further evidence that most samples giving reactive ELISA results are false positives can be seen from gender-specific reactivity rates for the first nine months of testing. Among donations from females 0.29% were repeatedly reactive; the rate in donations from males was 0.28%. Yet, the rate of Western blot positive samples from men was 0.05% compared to 0.01% for women.

Shortly after the first ELISA kits for anti-HTLV-III were licensed, a joint study between the American Red Cross Blood Services, Atlanta Region, and the CDC was undertaken to evaluate the performance of production-lot kits in a blood donor population (Ward et al 1986). The test evaluated, the Abbott ELISA, has been used to screen the great majority of USA blood donors through mid-1986. Samples from Atlanta donors who were non-reactive, initially reactive and repeatedly reactive were further tested at CDC by the Abbott ELISA and Western blot, and they were cultured for HTLV-III. From 25 March 1985 through 31 July 1985, 67 190 donor units were screened at the Atlanta blood centre, of which 569 (0.85%) were initially reactive. Only 171 (0.25% of all donations) were repeatedly reactive. CDC received samples from 628 non-reactive, 306 initially reactive, and 150 repeatedly reactive donors. No samples from the first or second group were Western blot positive or culture positive. Repeatedly reactive samples were divided into three groups based on the ELISA sample to cutoff (S/CO) ratio. Weak reactives (S/CO < 3.0) numbered 86 (57.3%); there were 19 (12.7%) moderate reactives (S/CO > 3.0, but < 6.0), and 45 (30.0%) were strong reactives (S/CO > 6.0). Strongly reactive samples were more likely to be Western blot positive (84.4%) and culture positive (51.1%) than weakly or moderately reactive samples of which only 1.0% were Western blot positive and 1.9% culture positive. Two weakly reactive samples were Western blot negative but culture positive. Of all repeatedly reactive samples, 26.0% were Western blot positive and 16.7% were culture positive. Using these two criteria as indices of infection, 28% of blood donors with repeatedly reactive ELISA tests were judged infected. The prevalence of HTLV-III infection in this blood donor population was estimated at 0.07%.

CONFIRMATORY TESTING

From the outset of routine blood donor screening it was apparent that an additional test(s) would be necessary to confirm samples identified as positive by the ELISA screening tests. The need for a confirmatory test was based on the low expected prevalence of HTLV-III positive blood donors (Sarngadharan et al 1984) and the estimated sensitivities of the ELISA tests derived from the clinical trials which, on theoretical grounds (Griner et al 1981), made it likely that the predictive value of a positive test result would be quite low (< 20%). The Western blot method has become the de facto confirmatory assay, but IFA has also been successfully used in the same capacity. After briefly describing each method, their respective merits and drawbacks will be covered in this section.

In essence, the Western blot test is an indirect antiglobulin assay which uses viral antigens produced in cell culture. The viral antigens are initially separated using polyacrylamide gel electrophoresis and then electrophoretically transferred to nitrocellulose sheets in a second step. The sheets are cut into strips which are then used as a source of separated viral antigens for the assay. A dilution of the donor's serum or plasma is incubated with the nitrocellulose strip containing the separated viral antigens. Excess unbound serum is removed by washing and an enzyme-labeled anti-human IgG conjugate is applied to the strip. After further incubation and washing, the strip is incubated with a substrate. The reaction is stopped by a final wash. If the sample contains antibody to HTLV-III coloured areas will developed on the strip identifying antibody complexes with viral antigens of different molecular weights. Major viral antigens are found at the following molecular weights (X 1000): 15/17, 24, 31, 41, 53/55, 65, 120, and 160. Because p 24 and gp 41 are respectively the major core and envelope proteins of the virus, their detection, with or without the other antigens, constitutes a positive test.

Most donor sera found positive in the ELISA screening test are non-reactive in the Western blot test (> 80%). Samples reactive by Western blot usually detect several viral antigens and are thus readily interpreted. Donors with these typical patterns are likely to be HTLV-III positive (Ward et al 1986). Less easy to interpret is the minority of samples which yield single lines on Western blot, e.g. p 15/17, p 24, or p 55, or combinations of lines not including p 24 or gp 41. Preliminary data indicate that some of these atypical blots are from persons who are truly positive. 6 of 11 donors who were positive for p 24 alone were virus culture-positive in a study conducted by the CDC and the Atlanta Red Cross blood centre (Ward et al 1986), and two virus-positive donors with atypical Western blots, one with p 24 alone and one with p 51 and p 65, were reported from an FDA study (Petricianni et al 1985).

The difficulty of interpreting atypical blot patterns, the subjective readout, and the technical demands of the assay have led to the search for easier methods of confirming ELISA-positive samples. IFA has proven to be a suitable alternative method for this purpose.

HTLV-III-infected and uninfected H9 cells are acetone-fixed on slides. A dilution of donor serum is applied to both infected and uninfected cells. After incubation, unbound serum is washed away and an anti-human IgG conjugated with fluorescein isothiocyanate is added to the test and control cells. Following incubation the excess conjugate is removed, the slides are mounted, and the cells are observed with a fluorescence microscope. Characteristic staining patterns are observed with serum samples containing antibody to HTLV-III (Sandstrom et al 1985). Samples with antibody to H9 cells can be readily differentiated from anti-HTLV-III containing sera by viewing the uninfected control cells. Although the readout is subjective, the experienced laboratory worker can readily detect anti-HTLV-III positive sera and reliably distinguish them from samples with anti-cell antibody.

Two studies have shown excellent correlation between IFA and Western blot and support the use of IFA as a confirmatory test for ELISA reactive samples (Sandstrom et al 1985, Gallo et al 1986). Though less complicated than the Western blot technically, IFA also relies on subjective interpretation and does require equipment not found in many smaller blood centres. Hence, a simpler confirmatory test with an objective readout is still a desirable objective.

Once the initial sample is confirmed as positive, it is imperative that an additional sample from the same donor be tested to avoid the possibility of sample error before what is perceived as an ominous result is reported to a volunteer donor. The management of these donors may be the most difficult aspect of HTLV-III screening.

PROBLEMS WITH HTLV-III ELISA TESTS

Because HTLV-III kits were designed to screen blood and plasma donors to prevent transfusion-transmitted AIDS, cutoffs for each test kit were set conservatively to maximize sensitivity, inevitably at the expense of some specificity. Moreover, data generated in the prelicensure period by the manufacturers indicated that the prevalence of HTLV-III antibody in donors would be low, perhaps 1% or less. Even though all seven licensed kits have very good sensitivity and specificity, the predictive value of positive test results in this low prevalence setting will be very low, i.e. most positive test results will be false positives. Therefore, it is not surprising that more than 20 000 USA blood donors are now on deferral lists because of false positive ELISA test results.

All manufacturers' tests show a disparity between initially reactive and repeatedly reactive samples. Such nonrepeatable reactives are likely to be due to technical errors which can arise from inaccurate sample dilutions, incorrect incubation times or temperatures, inadequate washing and splashing of conjugate. Repeatedly reactive false positives can arise with samples that are contaminated with microorganisms, have been heat-treated, or freeze-thawed numerous times.

The fact that all seven licensed kits are antiglobulin assays has undoubtedly contributed to the false positive problem because any immunoglobulin which binds to the solid phase, whether specifically or non-specifically, will produce a positive test result. Despite efforts to purify HTLV-III antigen preparations, the fact that the virus matures by budding through the cell membrane makes the removal of cellular contaminants very difficult. Thus, test design and the nature of the virus maturation process are both likely to lead to so-called biological false positives. Repeatedly reactive donors are more likely to be of this kind.

Testing of ELISA reactive, Western blot negative samples detected by one kit with other licensed ELISA kits has shown that a majority are not reactive despite the fact that six of seven manufacturers use HTLV-III grown in the H9 cell line and similar virus purification protocols (Holland et al 1985, Fang et al 1986).

Two studies have implicated HLA antibodies as one source of biological false positive ELISA results (Kühnl et al 1985, Sayers et al 1986). The first found that sera from multiparous women having anti-HLA Class I and II specificities were reactive in one licensed test. The second study found HLA antibodies directed against HLA antigens in eight of 11 women donors giving false positive ELISA test results. Seven of the eight had antibodies against Class II antigens including DR4 and DQw3. The latter antigens are also expressed on the H9 cell line.

Increased rates of false positive ELISA results have also been reported from patients with autoimmune diseases, e.g. rheumatoid arthritis, systemic lupus erythematosus and connective tissue diseases (Britz et al 1986).

Concerns have been recently raised about the sensitivity of ELISA kits. Sources of false negative test results are persons who have been recently infected and have not yet mounted an antibody response. The time from exposure to seroconversion in most infected individuals is two to three months (Ho et al 1985, Esteban et al 1985, Ludlam et al 1985); however, some persons may remain seronegative for longer periods or may not seroconvert at all. Antibody-negative, virus-positive asymptomatic risk group members have been documented in two studies (Salahuddin et al 1984, Mayer et al 1986). A total of five persons were described, all of whom were sexual partners of patients with AIDS or AIDS-related complex or had more than 100 lifetime homosexual partners. These virus-positive subjects were not followed longitudinally; therefore, it is unknown whether they were in the process of seroconverting or whether they represent antibody-negative carriers.

Limited data suggest that currently licensed tests differ in their ability to detect recent seroconversion (Ulstrup et al 1986, Saah 1986). The latter study found discrepant ELISA results on samples from homosexual and bisexual men which were frequently positive only for antibody to p 24, the major core protein, by Western blot. 30 samples in this category were selected and tested with five of the seven licensed ELISA kits. DuPont and Genetic Systems detected the same 25, Abbott 13, ElectroNucleonics 4, and Bionetics 2. Later samples from the 30 study subjects which contained both anti-core (p 24) and anti-envelope (gp 41) antibodies were detected with greater accuracy by all manufacturers.

We have studied 17 volunteer donors who have been repeatedly reactive by ELISA on at least one occasion. Parallel testing with ELISA kits from Abbott, DuPont, and Genetic Systems has been performed on 56 samples from these individuals. Sixteen of the donors have been confirmed positive by the presence of both p 24 and gp 41 in at least one sample. The remaining donor was nonreactive by all three ELISA screening methods on three samples taken at six-month intervals; however, Western blot detected bands in the p 15/17 region in each of the three ELISA-negative samples.

A fourth sample drawn six months later was positive by all three ELISA methods and bands at p 15/17, 31, 53/55 were detected by Western blot. Only one of the 56 samples gave discordant ELISA results. A seroconversion sample that was confirmable by Western blot (bands in regions p 15/17, p 24 and gp 41) was reactive by both DuPont and Genetic Systems but nonreactive by the Abbott ELISA. A sample taken from this donor seven months later was reactive by all three kits. The explanation for differential ELISA test sensitivity on samples from recent seroconverters may relate to different proportions of envelope and core proteins found in a given manufacturer's HTLV-III antigen preparation or the conditions under which the antigen is applied to the solid phase.

Because all HTLV-III-based assays use anti-human IgG conjugates (heavy and light chain specific), the inability to detect IgM class antibody efficiently may give rise to some false negative results. Whatever their origins may be, false negative test results must be minimized. The first report of transfusion-associated AIDS in a blood recipient since the advent of routine donor screening for HTLV-III has appeared recently (CDC 1986b). The implicated donor was a homosexual man who seroconverted to anti-HTLV-III between his August 1985 and November 1985 donations. Platelets from the August donation went to a 60-year-old man who was clinically normal but reactive for HTLV-III antibody in February 1986. This episode highlights the importance of test sensitivity in preventing the spread of transfusion-transmitted HTLV-III infection. Fortunately, such cases are likely to be extremely rare unless self-deferral guidelines are wantonly disregarded or HTLV-III infection spreads rapidly into segments of the population not included in the currently recognized risk groups.

HTLV-III ANTIBODY TESTING IN THE UK

The rate and extent to which AIDS has spread in Europe has lagged behind the USA. As of November 1983, 267 cases had been reported from Europe compared to 2803 in the USA (CDC 1983b); 24 cases were reported from the UK at this time. By October 1984 the 559 cases from Europe included 17 haemophiliacs and three transfusion recipients. Three of the haemophiliacs were included among the 88 cases reported from the UK (CDC 1985b). By 1986, only five patients with transfusion-associated AIDS had been reported from the UK, two of whom had received their transfusions outside the country (CDC 1986a). Screening of blood donors for anti-HTLV-III had shown none of 1042 to be seropositive in 1984 (Cheinsong-Popov et al 1984). Nevertheless, the long incubation period for transfusion AIDS and the likelihood of the continued spread of HTLV-III infection prompted the initiation of a programme to evaluate tests (Mortimer et al 1985) and implement screening at Blood Transfusion Centres in the UK.

Five commercial kits were evaluated at the Public Health Laboratory Service, Colindale, including Abbott, ElectroNucleonics, Litton Bionetics,

Organon Teknika, and Wellcome. They were compared against a panel of 360 sera from blood donors, risk group members and problem patients, i.e. patients whose sera are likely to give false positive results. Two kits, Organon and Wellcome, discriminated between reactive and non-reactive sera most clearly and were selected for use at blood transfusion services because they were rapid, reproducible, and convenient to use. The Organon test is a sandwich-type antiglobulin assay, whereas the Wellcome test is a competitive enzyme immunoassay, a method with inherently greater specificity.

Kits from Organon Teknika and Wellcome were further evaluated at Regional Transfusion Centres in North London and Manchester where they proved to be suitable for large-scale screening. During the evaluation period, alternative testing sites were established to provide access to HTLV-III testing for persons who were not blood donors, and arrangements were made to have repeatedly reactive samples confirmed by other methods at Public Health Laboratory Service Laboratories in England and Wales and University Laboratories in Scotland.

Table 7.3   Anti-HTLV-III screening in the UK.

Manufacturer (Donations Screened)	Initially Reactive (%)	Repeatedly Reactive (%)	Confirmed Positive (%)
Wellcome (778 000)	3705 (0.48)	69 (0.009)	14 (0.002)
Organon (274 000)	1713 (0.62)	403 (0.147)	5 (0.002)

Nation-wide (UK) testing commenced on 14 October 1985 at all Regional Blood Transfusion Centres. Organon kits were used at five centers; 16 chose the Wellcome test. Results accumulated after screening 1 052 000 donations are presented in Table 7.3. The Wellcome test detected lower rates of initial and repeat reactive samples than the Organon test. The greater specificity of the competitive assay is apparent in the higher % of repeatedly reactive samples which could be confirmed ($14/69 = 20\%$) relative to the sandwich assay ($5/403 = 1\%$). Though based on smaller numbers, the rate of confirmed positive donations in the UK (0.002%) is tenfold lower than current rates in the USA (0.02%). Both tests selected for use in the UK are generating far fewer initially reactive and repeatedly reactive samples than USA tests. Some of the disparity could be attributable to differences in the respective donor populations, but it is more likely to relate to the particular ELISA kits used for screening.

FUTURE DIRECTIONS IN HTLV-III TESTING

The accumulating evidence seems to indicate the need for improvements in sensitivity of some ELISA tests, particularly in detecting early seroconversions. This may be accomplished by changes in the quantity or quality of the antigens used, e.g. recombinant core or envelope proteins may be used to supplement or supplant cell-culture produced antigens. Until more is known about the natural history of HTLV-III infection, it will be impossible to custom design tests to include the most useful spectrum of antigens to maximize test sensitivity. Whether current tests need to be supplemented with IgM-specific conjugates requires further exploration.

Second generation tests, i.e. those having greater sensitivity and specificity, are being developed through the use of recombinant proteins, monoclonal antibodies, and novel solid phase supports and detection systems. The feasibility of detecting HBsAg and anti-HTLV-III with a single test is also being explored.

A prototype HTLV-III antigen test has been described (McDougal et al 1985). A second antigen test has detected antigen in 11 of 35 longitudinally followed homosexual and bisexual men with multiple male sex partners all of whom seroconverted. Five of these had detectable antigen prior to seroconversion, two simultaneously and the remainder from two to nine months afterward (Goudsmit et al 1986). The same test detected antigen in two recipients of blood prior to their antibody seroconversion (Alter & Esteban 1986). Antigen tests can be used to further explore the natural history of HTLV-III infection. Such tests, used in combination with HTLV-III DNA probes and virus culture, will enable a true assessment of the frequency of potentially infectious, antibody-negative blood donors to be made.

Specificity problems encountered with sandwich-type antiglobulin assays will be resolved by using more highly purified cell-culture-grown virus or recombinant proteins. Changes in assay design could also remedy this problem, e.g. using competitive rather than sandwich assays, as the UK experience has proven. Even with improved screening tests, the need for more reliable confirmatory tests to replace Western blot and IFA remains. Ideally such tests would be simple to perform and incorporate an objective readout. A competitive binding assay employing recombinant HTLV-III proteins is now being used in Europe; it seems to possess most of the desired characteristics of a definitive confirmatory test.

Recently, two new human retroviruses have been discovered in Africa (Kanki et al 1986), one of which is associated with AIDS (Clavel et al 1986). Sera from persons infected with these viruses react weakly with HTLV-III or LAV, respectively. These discoveries, along with the previous documentation of the genetic heterogeneity of HTLV- III (Wong-Staal et al 1985, Hahn et al 1986), make it clear that current HTLV-III tests will have to be continuously monitored for adequacy.

CURRENT ASSESSMENT OF ELISA SCREENING FOR ANTI-HTLV-III

It is always hoped, perhaps unrealistically, that a test can be developed that will be perfect – one that will accurately predict and guarantee the safety of each and every blood transfusion without ever being falsely positive or falsely negative. None of the present screening tests for anti-HTLV-III is that perfect test. This does not mean, however, that these tests are unlikely to be useful in greatly reducing the incidence of AIDS associated with transfusion, particularly when combined with other measures.

AIDS attributable to blood and blood component transfusion from single donors makes up a small proportion of the AIDS cases in the USA. As of June 1986, there have been 351 cases (1.7% of the total 21 420) in adults and adolescents, and 45 cases (14.7% of the total 306) in children less than 13 years old. Since March of 1983, donors who fall into high risk categories have been asked to refrain from donating for transfusion purposes. Guidelines as to who is considered a high risk donor have been modified over this time but as of September 1985, any male who has had any homosexual involvement since 1977 has been included in the high risk category (CDC 1985c). HTLV-III antibody testing was begun in March 1985 and was in use by every collecting organization in the USA by the summer of 1985. The transfusion associated AIDS cases presented in Table 7.4 represent the composite effects of the policy of donor exclusion, the changing rate of infection in the donor base, and the lengthy incubation phase in recipients until they develop AIDS as defined by the CDC. Since both the median and mean duration from transfusion to clinical AIDS are about 20 months, the case stabilization apparent in the 1986 data is not likely to reflect, as yet, any significant benefit from HTLV-III antibody screening. However, the policy of donor exclusion has had the effect of holding the rate of transfusion-associated AIDS to a straight line progression for the past year and one-half at a time when there has been a substantial increase in the percentage of serologically positive people in the high risk categories.

Table 7.4   Transfusion-associated AIDS in the United States from CDC AIDS surveillance reports.

	Prior to 14 Jan 84	14 Jan 84 to 13 Jan 85	14 Jan 85 to 13 Jan 86	14 Jan 86 to 6 June86
Adults	34	56	171	90
Children	6	6	21	12

It is important that individuals in high risk categories continue to be dissuaded from being blood donors and that, as different risk groups become known, they and their sexual partners be added to the interdicted groups. This is particularly imperative since the present screening test detects an antibody response to infection and is not a specific assay of infectivity; it is therefore bound – as has already occurred in one incident – to allow the transfusion of an infectious unit from a serologically negative high risk donor.

Table 7.5 Will the HTLV-III antibody test be effective?

3 million recipients/year with survival into third year
9 million units/year transfused to survivors
3600 potentially infected units tranfused prior to screening
180 expected AID cases at 5% estimated
Actual number of AIDS cases for 1985 = 192
Projected number of AIDS cases for 1986 = 240

Are the screening tests for anti-HTLV-III presently used likely to eliminate the risk of AIDS transmission? If one expects absolutely no risk, the answer is no. But if one assumes that the groups at high risk will for the most part continue to refrain from donating, then we can estimate the benefit to be derived from screening. At the moment it appears that there are, depending upon geographic area, between 0.2 and 10.0 antibody positive individuals per 10 000 donors with an average of 4 per 10 000 (0.04%) established in the first million tested in the USA. If one assumes that every positive unit will infect a recipient, then some estimates concerning the magnitude of transfusion-associated AIDS resulting from the pre-screening era can be made (Table 7.5).

Based on our transfusion records for 1983–85, we have determined that about 3% of the patients are transfused with more than 10 units of red cell-containing products in less than 24 hours. This group uses 12–13% of the blood and 20–25% of the platelets. The remaining 75–80% of the platelets are given to another 5% of the patients for haematological disorders. They also use about 10% of the red cell products. We can assume that the vast majority of these people do not survive for more than two years.

Using the foregoing information and the fact that approximately 40% of all transfused patients are over 65 years of age, we have estimated the efficacy of donor screening based on the following assumptions. Transfusion-associated AIDS will be found most likely in recipients of red cell and whole blood units. 75% of the patients receiving these units will be alive in the third year after transfusion and will have received an average of 3 units of blood. If we assume that there are 3 million patients yearly in this category, 3600 would have received potentially infected units (0.04% of 9 million) during each year prior to testing. Given the mean and median for transfusion-associated cases reported until now has been approximately two years, the bulk of the 1985 and 1986 cases would have been exposed in 1983 and 1984. As screening was begun in mid-1985, these new cases reported by mid-1987 should only have incubation phases of over two years if the screening tests are perfect. If the screening tests are only 95% effective then there should be 9–10 cases with incubation periods of less than two years reported between mid-1987 and 1988. The epidemiological data that develop in that year will allow us to ascertain the efficacy of the screening tests. We anticipate that there will only be a few such cases but would not expect a significant drop in the number of transfusion-associated cases reported annually until 1988 or 1989.

Acknowledgement

The authors are indebted to Dr J. A. J. Barbara of the North London Blood Transfusion Centre at Edgware for much of the information concerning the HTLV-III donor screening programme in the UK. The authors also thank Mr Laurence H. Parks for his excellent editorial assistance in the preparation of this manuscript.

REFERENCES

Alter H, Esteban J 1986 HTLV-III infection in asymptomatic blood donors. Presented at the National Institutes of Health Consensus Development Conference on 'Impact of routine HTLV-III antibody testing on public health,' July 7–9, 1986

Ammann A J, Cowan M J, Wara D W et al 1983 Acquired immunodeficiency in an infant: possible transmission by means of blood products. Lancet 1: 956–958

Barré-Sinoussi F, Chermann J C, Rey F et al 1983 Isolation of a T-lymphotropic retrovirus from a patient at risk for acquired immune deficiency syndrome (AIDS). Science 220: 868–871

Britz J A, Zimmerman D H, Mundon F K et al 1986 The HTLV-III ELISA: a sensitive and specific test for the detection of antibodies to human T-lymphotropic virus. Luiz de la Maza (ed) The International Symposium on Medical Virology, Anaheim, California. Lawrence Erlbaum Associates, Hillsdale, New Jersey (in press)

Centers for Disease Control 1981 Pneumocystis pneumonia – Los Angeles. Morbidity and Mortality Weekly Report 30: 250–252

Centers for Disease Control 1982 Pneumocystis carinii pneumonia among persons with hemophilia A. Morbidity and Mortality Weekly Report 31: 365–367

Centers for Disease Control 1983a Prevention of acquired immune deficiency syndrome (AIDS): Report of inter-agency recommendations. Morbidity and Mortality Weekly Report 32: 101–104

Centers for Disease Control 1983b Acquired immunodeficiency syndrome (AIDS) – Europe. Morbidity and Mortality Weekly Report 32: 610–611

Centers for Disease Control 1985a Provisional Public Health Service inter-agency recommendations for screening donated blood and plasma for antibody to the virus causing acquired immunodeficiency syndrome. Morbidity and Mortality Weekly Report 34: 1–5

Centers for Disease Control 1985b Update: acquired immunodeficiency syndrome – Europe. Morbidity and Mortality Weekly Report 34: 21–31

Centers for Disease Control 1985c Update: Revised Public Health Service definition of persons who should refrain from donating blood and plasma – United States. Morbidity and Mortality Weekly Report 34: 547–548

Centers for Disease Control 1986a Update: acquired immunodeficiency syndrome – Europe. Morbidity and Mortality Weekly Report 35: 35–46

Centers for Disease Control 1986b Transfusion-associated human T-lymphotropic virus type III/lymphadenopathy-associated virus infection from a seronegative donor – Colorado. Morbidity and Mortality Weekly Report. 35: 389–391

Cheingsong-Popov R, Weiss R A, Dalgleish A et al 1984 Prevalence of antibody to human T-lymphotropic virus type III in AIDS and AIDS-risk patients in Britain. Lancet 2: 477–480

Clavel F, Guétard D, Brun-Vézinet F et al 1986 Isolation of a new human retrovirus from West African patients with AIDS. Science 233: 343–346

Coffin J, Haase A, Levy J A et al 1986 Human immunodeficiency viruses. Science 232:697

Culliton B J 1984 Crash development of AIDS test nears goal. Science 225: 1128–1131

Essex M, McLane M F, Lee T H et al 1983 Antibodies to cell membrane antigens associated with human T-cell leukemia virus in patients with AIDS. Science 220: 859–862

Esteban J I, Shih J W-K, Tai C-C et al 1985 Importance of Western blot analysis in predicting infectivity of anti-HTLV-III/LAV positive blood. Lancet 2: 1083–1086

Fang C T, Darr F, Kleinman S et al 1986 Relative specificity of enzyme-linked immunosorbent assays for antibodies to human T-cell lymphotropic virus, type III, and their relationship to Western blotting. Transfusion 26: 208–209

Gallo D, Diggs, J L, Shell, G R et al 1986 Comparison of detection of antibody to the acquired immune deficiency syndrome virus by enzyme immunoassay, immunofluorescence, and Western blot methods. Journal of Clinical Microbiology 23: 1049–1051

Gallo R C, Sarin P S, Gelmann E P et al 1983 Isolation of human T-cell leukemia virus in acquired immune deficiency syndrome (AIDS). Science 220: 865–867

Gallo R C, Salahuddin S Z, Popovic M et al 1984 Frequent detection and isolation of cytopathic retroviruses (HTLV-III) from patients with AIDS and at risk for AIDS. Science 224: 500–502

Goudsmit J, de Wolfe F, Paul D A et al 1986 Expression of human immunodeficiency virus antigen (HIV-Ag) in serum and cerebrospinal fluid during acute and chronic infection. Lancet 2: 177–180

Griner P F, Mayewski R J, Mushlin Al et al 1981 Selection and interpretation of diagnostic tests and procedures. Annals of Internal Medicine 94 (part 2): 565–567

Hahn B H, Shaw G M, Taylor M E et al 1986 Genetic variation in HTLV-III/LAV over time in patients with AIDS or at risk for AIDS. Science 232: 1548–1553

Ho D D, Sarngadharan M G, Resnick L et al 1985 Primary human T-lymphotropic virus type III infection. Annals of Internal Medicine. 103: 880–883

Holland P V, Richards C A, Teghtmeyer J R et al 1985 Anti-HTLV-III testing of blood donors: reproducibility and confirmability of commercial test kits. Transfusion 25: 395–397

Kanki P J, Barin F, M'Boup S et al 1986 New human T-lymphotropic retrovirus related to simian T-lymphotropic virus type III (STLV-III$_{AGM}$) Science 232: 238–243

Kühnl P, Seidl S, Holzberger G 1985 HLA DR4 antibodies cause positive HTLV-III antibody ELISA results. Lancet 1: 1222–1223

Kuritsky J N, Rastogi S C, Faich G A et al 1986 Results of nationwide screening of blood and plasma for antibodies to human T-cell lymphotrophic III virus, type III. Transfusion 26: 205–207

Ludlam C A, Tucker J, Steel C M, et al 1985 Human T-lymphotropic virus type III (HTLV-III) infection in seronegative haemophiliacs after transfusion of factor VIII. Lancet. 2: 233–256

Mayer K H, Stoddard A M, McCusker J et al 1986 Human T-lymphotropic virus type III in high-risk, antibody-negative homosexual men. Annals of Internal Medicine. 104: 194–196

McDougal J S, Cort S P, Kennedy M S et al 1985 Immunoassay for the detection and quantitation of infectious human retrovirus, lymphadenopathy-associated virus (LAV). Journal of Immunological Methods 76: 171–183

Mortimer P P, Parry J V, Mortimer J Y 1985 Which anti-HTLV-III/LAV assays for screening and confirmatory testing? Lancet 2: 873–877

Petricianni J C, Seto B, Wells M, et al 1985 An analysis of serum samples positive for HTLV-III antibodies. New England Journal of Medicine 313: 47–48

Popovic M, Sarngadharan M G, Read E et al 1984 Detection, isolation, and continuous production of cytopathic retroviruses (HTLV-III) from patients with AIDS and pre-AIDS. Science 224: 497–500

Saah A J 1986 ELISA sensitivity in early HTLV-III/LAV infection. Presented at the National Institutes of Health Consensus Development Conference on 'Impact of routine HTLV-III antibody testing on public health.' July 7–9

Salahuddin S Z, Groopman J E, Markham P D et al 1984 HTLV-III in symptom-free seronegative persons. Lancet 2: 1418–1420

Sandler S G 1986 Testing blood donors for HTLV-III antibodies: The American Red Cross experience. Presented at the National Institutes of Health Consensus Development Conference on 'Impact of routine HTLV-III antibody testing on public health.' July 7–9

Sandstrom E G, Schooley R T, Ho D D et al 1985 Detection of human anti-HTLV-III antibodies by indirect immunofluorescence using fixed cells. Transfusion 25: 308–312

Sarngadharan M G, Popovic M, Bruch L et al 1984 Antibodies reactive with human T-lymphotropic retroviruses (HTLV-III) in the serum of patients with AIDS. Science 224: 506–508

Sayers M H, Beatty P G, Hansen J A 1986 HLA antibodies as a cause of false-positive reactions in screening enzyme immunoassays for antibodies to human T-lymphotropic virus type III. Transfusion 26: 113–115

Schorr J B, Berkowitz A, Cumming P D et al 1985 Prevalence of HTLV-III antibody in American blood donors. New England Journal of Medicine 313: 384–385

Ulstrup J C, Skaug K, Figenschau K J et al 1986 Sensitivity of Western blotting (compared with ELISA and immunofluorescence) during seroconversion after HTLV-III infection. Lancet 1: 1151–1152

Ward J W, Grindon A J, Feorino P M et al 1986 Laboratory and epidemiologic evaluation of an enzyme immunoassay for antibodies to HTLV-III. Journal of the American Medical Association 256: 357–361

Wong-Staal F, Shaw G M, Hahn B H et al 1985 Genomic diversity of human T-lymphotropic virus type III (HTLV-III). Science 229: 759–762

L. R. Sehgal   A. L. Rosen   S. A. Gould
H. L. Sehgal   R. DeWoskin   G. S. Moss

8

Haemoglobin solutions as red cell substitutes

INTRODUCTION

The attempt to develop a temporary red cell substitute, based on haemoglobin, has spanned many decades with limited success.

With one exception, all haemoglobin based red cell substitutes are acellular. These solutions can be defined as colloid solutions like albumin, dextran or hydroxyethyl starch, but having the important added property of being able to carry oxygen.

A red cell substitute, in order to be clinically useful, has to be both safe and effective. Furthermore, it has to fulfill some additional logistic requirements. It should have an extended shelf life. It should be temperature stable, preferably at ambient conditions. It should not have the typing and cross-matching requirements of blood. It should be functional in terms of oxygen loading and unloading in room air. When administered it should provide additional oxygen carrying capacity, for a reasonable length of time.

From a biochemical point-of-view an ideal acellular oxygen carrier should have a normal oxygen carrying capacity. The oxygen loading and unloading characteristics, defined by the P_{50}, should again be comparable to the haemoglobin within the red cell. Furthermore, any chemical modification to improve the P_{50} of the haemoglobin and normalize the oxygen carrying capacity should not shield the binding sites for oxygen and reduce the binding capacity. Finally, any modification that increases the rate of autoxidation would significantly reduce the benefits of the chemical alterations, by lowering the oxygen carrying capacity and by increasing the oxygen affinity.

Several approaches have evolved over the past decades for the preparation of a haemoglobin solution that is essentially free of red cell membrane debris or 'stroma-free haemoglobin' (SFH). In this chapter, an attempt will be made to provide an overview of the progress made with SFH to date and its current status.

128

BACKGROUND

There are numerous papers describing the injection of haemoglobin solutions in man (Sellards et al 1916, Amberson 1934). None of these early studies, however, explored the therapeutic utility of SFH in the correction of acute anaemia (Amberson et al 1934). The first important clinical study that utilized haemoglobin solution in the treatment of shock was that by Amberson et al (1949). Fourteen patients were studied. They received significant amounts of haemoglobin in multiple injections. The important observations made included a vasoconstrictive activity of the solution, associated with a temporary diminution of renal function. All adverse effects were transient and there was no mortality associated with the infusions. None of the animal studies preceding this clinical evaluation predicted this human response to haemoglobin.

The adverse effects noted were attributed to stromal contaminations by subsequent investigators (Rabiner et al 1967, Birndorf et al, 1971, Moss et al 1973). The haemoglobin solution used by Amberson et al (1949) was prepared by ether or toluene extraction of stromal lipids. The level of stromal lipids in their solution was not stated.

Rabiner et al (1967) developed an alternate method of preparation that involved gentle osmotic lysis (Dodge et al 1963) followed by centrifugation and filtration. This method of preparation resulted in significantly lower levels of stromal lipids. Several other methods of preparation of 'stroma-free' haemoglobin solutions have been reported that involve osmotic lysis and filtration (Sehgal et al 1983a), crystallization (Canan et al 1942, DeVenuto et al 1977), or acid precipitation (Hamilton et al 1947) of stroma. All of the current procedures appear to render the haemoglobin solution essentially stroma-free based on the chemical determination of phospholipids. Furthermore, none of these preparations show any effect on coagulation as measured by PT and APTT. The general properties of SFH are shown in Table 8.1.

Table 8.1 Characteristics of stroma-free haemoglobin.

	SFH	Whole blood
[Hb]	6–8 g/dl	12–14 gm/dl
O_2 carrying capacity	8.0–11.0 vol %	16–19 vol %
Binding coefficient	1.30 cc O_2/g Hb	1.30 cc O_2-gHb
P_{50} (pCO_2 = 40 torr; pH = 7.40)	12–14 torr	26–28 torr
Methaemoglobin	<2%	<1%
Colloid osmotic pressure	18–25 torr	18–25 torr
Osmolarity	290–310 mOsm	290–310 mOsm
Total phospholipid	0.4 mg/dl	
Viscosity	1.6 cp (8 gm/dl)	3.2 cp

PHYSIOLOGY OF O$_2$ TRANSPORT BY SFH

Haemoglobin solution irrespective of the specific method of preparation will not contain 2,3,diphosphoglycerate (2,3,DPG) or any other organic phosphates present in the red cell. The loss of the modulating effect of 2,3,DPG on the O$_2$ haemoglobin dissociation curve results in a significant decrease in the P$_{50}$ of the solution compared to that of fresh blood (Fig. 8.1). Furthermore, the requirement to be iso-oncotic with plasma results in a 6–8 g% haemoglobin concentration (Fig. 8.2). It was thus not clear if a haemoglobin solution with half the normal oxygen carrying capacity and with a significantly increased affinity for oxygen would be able to deliver adequate amounts of oxygen to the tissues. This was tested in adult baboons.

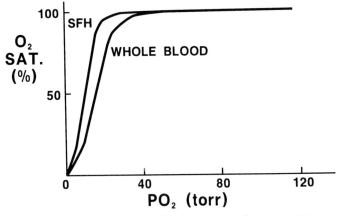

Fig. 8.1 O$_2$ dissociation curves for whole blood and stroma-free haemoglobin solution (SFH). Loss of DPG in SFH causes increased O$_2$ affinity.

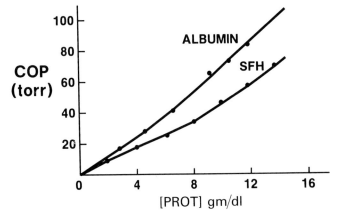

Fig. 8.2 Colloid osmotic pressure (COP) of albumin solution and stroma-free haemoglobin solution (SFH).

Nine animals underwent total exchange transfusion with haemoglobin solution, while nine control animals underwent exchange transfusion with dextran 70 (Moss et al 1976). All animals given haemoglobin solution survived to zero haematocrit. In contrast, all nine control animals died at haematocrit levels of approximately 5%.

The dextran-treated animals responded to isovolemic anaemia by an increase in cardiac output, an increase in oxygen extraction, and a decrease in mixed venous oxygen pressure ($P\bar{v}o_2$). The haemoglobin-treated animals developed only small changes in oxygen consumption at zero haematocrit when compared to baseline levels. The maintenance of near normal oxygen consumption at zero haematocrit was achieved primarily through the mechanism of increased oxygen extraction leading to low $P\bar{v}o_2$ levels. The fact that oxygen consumption was essentially unchanged at zero haematocrit was remarkable, since a radical change in the circulation had occurred. Blood containing 12 gm of haemoglobin/dl with a P_{50} of 32 torr was acutely replaced with a haemoglobin solution of 7 gm/dl with a P_{50} of 12 torr. Also remarkable was the mechanism of maintenance of oxygen consumption at zero haematocrit. In view of the profound shift in the affinity state, an increase in cardiac output rather than an elevation in oxygen extraction would have been the expected response.

Our study in baboons confirmed what Mulder et al (1934) had shown to be true in cats. Though animals temporarily survive such a massive assault on their circulation, a number of questions were raised from this study. One question concerned the dramatic reduction in $P\bar{v}o_2$ to 20 torr in the haemoglobin-treated animals at zero haematocrit. The $P\bar{v}o_2$ is the tension at which oxygen unloads from the haemoglobin and is in equilibrium with the tissue PO_2. Such a low $P\bar{v}o_2$ was alarming to us and led us to attempt its correction.

NORMALIZATION OF MIXED VENOUS OXYGEN TENSION

Factors that affect $P\bar{v}o_2$ include an increase in oxygen consumption and a decrease in cardiac output, arterial saturation, haemoglobin mass, or affinity state. Our data indicated minimal changes in oxygen consumption, arterial saturation, and cardiac output and therefore could not account for the decline in $P\bar{v}o_2$. That left changes in haemoglobin mass and affinity state for further consideration. We examined affinity state changes first. Fig. 8.3 demonstrates how a leftward shift in the content curve could produce a decrease in the tension at which oxygen unloading occurs – the $P\bar{v}o_2$. This possibility was confirmed by Riggs et al (1973) who exchange transfused monkeys with high-affinity banked monkey blood. They noted no change in cardiac output or arteriovenous oxygen content difference (A-VDO$_2$). They did observe a significant decrease in $P\bar{v}o_2$. No data existed concerning the consequences of normalizing a leftward shifted curve.

Attempts to normalize P_{50} by the addition of 2,3,DPG to the haemo-

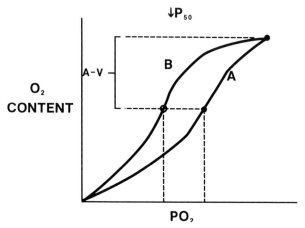

Fig. 8.3 O_2 content curves. Decrease in P_{50} from curve A to B will result in a fall in venous PO_2, if there is no change in (arterial-venous) $[O_2]$.

globin solution itself were unsuccessful, since the DPG rapidly disappears from the circulation after infusion. Benesch et al (1972), Greenberg et al (1977), and Sehgal et al (1981) described a chemical modification of the haemoglobin molecule by the addition of pyridoxal,5′-phosphate. Pyridoxylated haemoglobin, exhibits a P_{50} considerably higher than the P_{50} of unmodified haemoglobin. This modification allowed us to examine the $P\bar{v}o_2$ in animals exchange transfused with pyridoxylated haemoglobin.

Eight baboons were the test animals (Gould et al 1980). Four received unmodified haemoglobin (P_{50} = 12 torr), while four received pyridoxylated haemoglobin (P_{50} = 22 torr). A total exchange transfusion to zero haematocrit was carried out. The haemoglobin concentration of both solutions was approximately 7 g/dl. No important changes were noted following exchange

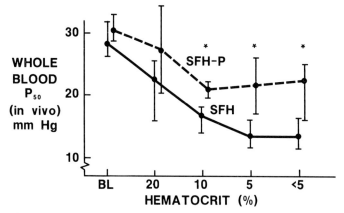

Fig. 8.4 Whole blood P_{50} during exchange transfusion with stroma-free haemoglobin solution (SFH) and pyridoxylated SFH (SFH-P). At haematocrits below 20%, the whole blood P_{50} was significantly higher in the presence of SFH-P.

transfusion in either group in oxygen consumption, cardiac output, or A-VDO$_2$. Figure 8.4 demonstrates that animals that underwent exchange transfusion with pyridoxylated haemoglobin developed significantly higher whole blood P$_{50}$ levels compared to those given unmodified haemoglobin when the haematocrit levels declined to 10%. From this point onward, P$\bar{v}$o$_2$ levels were substantially higher in the animals given pyridoxylated haemoglobin (Fig. 8.5).

These data illustrate two points. First, they confirm the concept that rightward shifts in the dissociation curve result in an increased P$\bar{v}$o$_2$, as long as cardiac output and A-VDO$_2$ remain constant. This is important since it allows for unloading to occur at a higher tissue PO$_2$. Second, the P$\bar{v}$o$_2$ level in the animals treated with pyridoxylated haemoglobin was still significantly lower than the 40–50 torr found in control animals. Thus we decided to search for other means to normalize the P$\bar{v}$o$_2$ in animals that underwent total exchange transfusion with haemoglobin solution. This led us to examine the quantitative relationship among changes in haemoglobin concentration, P$_{50}$ levels and P$\bar{v}$o$_2$.

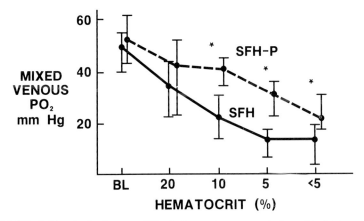

Fig. 8.5 Whole blood mixed venous PO$_2$ during exchange transfusion with SFH and SFH-P. At haematocrits below 20%, the venous PO$_2$ was significantly higher in the presence of SFH-P.

HAEMOGLOBIN CONCENTRATION, P$_{50}$, AND MIXED VENOUS OXYGEN TENSION

Little information existed concerning the relationship among changes in haemoglobin concentration, P$_{50}$, and the resultant P$\bar{v}$o$_2$ in animals receiving haemoglobin solutions. Such information could provide a clue concerning whether we should focus on further efforts to increase the P$_{50}$ of the haemoglobin solution or whether we should attempt to increase the haemoglobin concentration.

In this study 15 baboons underwent total exchange transfusion with pyridoxylated haemoglobin with a P_{50} of 21 torr and a haemoglobin concentration of 7 g/dl. (Gould et al 1982) The result involved simultaneous changes in both the recipient haemoglobin concentration and P_{50}. To assess the effect of each of these two variables on $P\bar{v}o_2$, we used a multiple linear regression model. The equation was as follows: $\triangle P\bar{v}o_2 = a . \triangle [Hb] + b . \triangle P_{50}$, where a is a coefficient for haemoglobin concentration and b is a coefficient for P_{50}. The results are shown in Table 8.2. The important results are a decrease in haemoglobin concentration of 6.5 g/dl and a decrease in P_{50} of 11.5 torr. These changes were associated with a decline in $P\bar{v}o_2$ of 29 torr.

Table 8.2 Calculated changes in mixed venous oxygen tension.

Variable	Average total change ($\triangle$)	Multiple regression coefficient	Contribution to $\triangle PvO_2$ (torr)
Haemoglobin concentration	−6.5	4.0	−26.0
P_{50}	−11.5	0.33	−3.8
		Total calculated $\triangle PvO_2$	−29.8
		vs.	
		Observed $\triangle$ PvO_2	−29.0

The coefficients of each variable (calculated from the equation) and the contributions of each variable to the change in $P\bar{v}o_2$ are shown in Table 8.2. The results show that the 6.5 g/dl decrease in haemoglobin cncentration produced a 26 torr decline in $P\bar{v}o_2$, whereas an 11.5 torr decline in P_{50} produced only a 3.8 torr decrease in $P\bar{v}o_2$. These changes clearly indicate that further efforts should be directed toward normalizing the haemoglobin concentration.

The advantages of haemoglobin solution with normal oxygen carrying capacity are self-evident. According to our data, the infusion of 12–15 g% solution should be associated with near normal $P\bar{v}o_2$ levels, even at zero haematocrit. The principal obstacle to normalization of haemoglobin concentration is the effect of an elevation in protein concentration on oncotic pressure.

The relationship between haemoglobin concentration and oncotic pressure is shown in Fig. 8.2. At haemoglobin concentrations of 7 g/dl, the oncotic pressure is similar to that of plasma-20 torr. In contrast, at haemoglobin levels of 15 gm/dl, oncotic pressure increases by more than 300%. The infusion of such a solution would theoretically produce large shifts of fluid from the extravascular space into the intravascular space. These changes are likely to be exceedingly harmful.

POLYMERIZED PYRIDOXYLATED HAEMOGLOBIN

Polymerization provides one approach to producing a nonanaemic haemo-globin solution with normal colloid osmotic pressure values (Bonsen et al 1977). The colloid osmotic pressure of any solution is proportional to the number of colloidal particles (Fig. 8.6). If a 15 g/dl solution of haemoglobin could be polymerized, the result would be a reduction in colloid osmotic pressure, while no change would occur in haemoglobin concentration (Fig. 8.7).

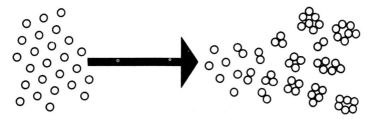

Fig. 8.6 Schematic representation of the polymerization of haemoglobin. There is a range of polymer sizes, and some haemoglobin tetramer escape polymerization.

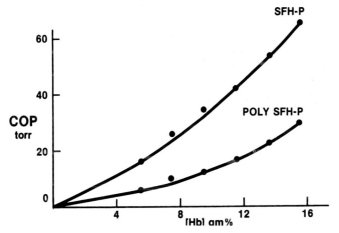

Fig. 8.7 Comparison of the colloid osmotic pressure (COP) of SFH-P and poly SFH-P. The SFH-P is hyperoncotic at [Hb] of 14 gm/dl, whereas the poly SFH-P is iso-oncotic at this concentration.

We were able to successfully polymerize pyridoxylated haemoglobin using glutaraldehyde as the cross-linking agent (Sehgal et al 1980). The end-point of the polymerization was a physiologically acceptable COP (20–30 torr).

Other investigators were also able to polymerize pyridoxylated haemo-globin (DeVenuto et al 1981, Keipert et al 1984, Kothe et al 1985) with comparable characteristics.

Table 8.3   Characteristics of polymerized pyridoxylated haemoglobin.

[Hb]	12–15 g/dl
Polymerization yield	75–85%
Molecular weight distribution	64–400 × 10^3 daltons
O_2 carrying capacity	16.7–21.0 vol%
Binding coefficient	1.30 cc O_2/g Hb
Methaemoglobin	<5%
Colloid osmotic pressure	15–20 torr
Osmolarity	290–310 mOsm
Total phospholipid[1]	<0.4 mg/dl
Viscosity	2–3 cp (8 g/dl)
Methaemoglobin reductase[2]	20–30% of normal

[1] Total phospholipid estimated by thin layer chromatography (Helena Laboratories test procedure)
[2] Methaemoglobin reductase activity assayed according to the method of Board et al 1981

The characteristics of this new solution are shown Table 8.3. The major points to emphasize are the normal oxygen-binding coefficient, the normal haemoglobin concentration, and the normal colloid osmotic pressure. The polymer yield ranges from 75–85% and the molecular weight distribution of polymers ranges from 120 000–600 000 (Sehgal et al 1983b).

The poly SFH-P thus made was first tested in rats (Sehgal et al 1980). Eight rats were divided into two groups of four each. The first group underwent total exchange transfusion with poly SFH-P. The second group received 5% albumin solution. All the control rats died at a haematocrit of approximately 5%. All the rats given poly SFH-P survived. This preliminary study suggested that the poly SFH-P was an effective O_2 carrier in the absence of red cells, despite its low P_{50}.

A second study was undertaken to determine the effect of polymerization on the intravascular retention of poly SFH-P. (Sehgal et al 1984). Previous reports have demonstrated a relatively short half-life of tetrameric haemoglobin of approximately 2–4 hours. Much of the tetramer is cleared by the kidneys, following dissociation into dimers and monomers. The half-life of the poly SFH-P was tested by infusion of 900 ml into adult baboons. Pyridoxylated haemoglobin served as the control solution. The poly SFH-P shows a striking increase in half-life to 38 hours, compared to about 6 hours for pyridoxylated haemoglobin (Fig. 8.8).

This first report on the characteristics and in vivo efficacy of poly SFH-P, has subsequently been confirmed by several other investigators. DeVenuto et al (1982) demonstrated a long term survival in rats following a 95% exchange transfusion with poly SFH-P infused at 7.5 g/dl. In constrast animals exchanged transfused with the tetrameric SFH died within five hours post exchange transfusion. Besides efficacy, this study also demonstrates a lack of gross toxicity of poly SFH-P. Feola et al (1983) documented the efficacy of a 7 g/dl bovine poly SFH-P in the resuscitation from haemorrhagic shock in rabbits. Up to 66% blood replacement was made in these studies. Animals resuscitated with unmodified human or bovine tetrameric haemoglobin died within two hours post resuscitation. In

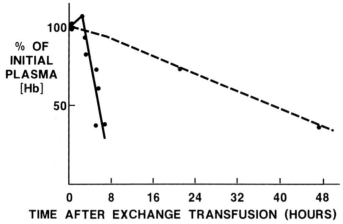

Fig. 8.8 Intra-vascular dwell time of SFH (solid line) and poly SFH-P (dashed line). The poly SFH-P has a plasma half-life approximately 10 times longer than SFH.

contrast animals resuscitated with the polymerized bovine SFH survived the resuscitation from haemorrhagic shock. Kiepert et al (1985) have also confirmed the efficacy of a 9 gm/dl poly SFH-P in a fully monitored haemorrhaged rats. They had a 75% long term survival (> 8 days) with poly SFH-P compared to 0% for the unmodified SFH and 83% for whole blood. Gould et al (1985) reported on a complete blood replacement (Hct $< 1\%$) in baboons with a 14 g/dl poly SFH-P. The haemodynamic and O_2 consumption data is shown in Table 8.4. No significant changes from baseline values were observed following total exchange transfusion with poly SFH-P.

Gould et al (1986) have also documented the efficacy of poly-SFH-P with respect to its contribution to total O_2 delivery and O_2 consumption in the presence of a significant red cell mass, since that is the most likely clinical setting. The methodology to assess the efficacy of any acellular oxygen carrier in the presence of red cells has been previously reported (Rosen et al 1983, 1986a). Using this technique, the contribution of O_2 delivery was approximately 40% at a haematocrit of 20%, 60% at a hematocrit of 10% and almost 80% at a haematocrit of 5%. Its contribution to O_2 consumption

Table 8.4 Haemodynamic and O_2 consumption data in baboons at baseline and following total exchange transfusion with poly SFH-P.

	Baseline	Poly SFH Hct < 1%
$\dot{V}O_2$ (cc/min)	60.1 ± 8.5	58.0 ± 4.8
MAP (torr)	138 ± 8	140 ± 8
HR (bpm)	114 ± 3	117 ± 10
CO (L/min)	1.63 ± 0.26	1.30 ± 0.2

was 20% at Hct = 20, 40% at Hct = 10 and 60% at Hct = 5%. Thus the poly SFH-P, despite its lower P_{50} (16–20 torr) compared to the baboon P_{50} of 32 torr made significant contributions to both O_2 delivery and consumption.

Polymerization of unmodified SFH has also been done using other polymerizing agents (Mok et al 1975, Morris et al 1977, Horowitz et al 1978). These approaches have not subsequently been pursued, with respect to safety and efficacy studies.

There are some reports of intramolecular cross-linking of haemoglobin with imidoesters (Horowitz et al 1978) or bifunctional pyridoxal phosphate (Benesch et al 1975). This approach may solve the problem of haemoglobinuria only, but would not normalize the O_2 carrying capacity.

Unmodified haemoglobin has been successfully cross-linked to dextran (Blumenstein et al 1978) albumin (Rozenberg et al 1978) polyethylene glycol (Ajisaka et al 1980), and hydroxyetheyl starch (Baldwin et al 1981). All these complexes result in a significant increase in intravascular half-life. But all of them have significantly below normal oxygen carrying capacity. Furthermore, all of them appear to have one or more undesirable physiologic characteristics with respect to COP, viscosity, and P_{50}. The benefit of these polymeric species over polymerized haemoglobin is not clear.

In summary, from the view point of the efficacy of oxygen transport, poly SFH-P appears to be the most promising candidate solution for further preclinical investigations.

BARRIERS TO CLINICAL TRIALS

So far we have reviewed the efficacy of haemoglobin solution with regard to oxygen transport. The next issue is safety. The predominant concern lies in the area of nephrotoxicity. Of secondary concern are issues of immunogenecity and immunosuppression.

Nephrotoxicity was reported in early studies following the infusion of haemoglobin solutions. Further investigations suggested that the stroma was the toxic factor, probably on the basis of thrombosis of the small renal vasculature (Rabiner et al 1968). Haemoglobin solution, relatively free of stroma, produced no deterioration in renal function following infusion in dogs. These findings were subsequently confirmed in monkeys, even in stressful circumstances of dehydration and shock (Birndorf et al 1970).

In 1978 Savitsky et al reported the results of a clinical safety trial in humans using stroma-free haemoglobin. Eight healthy male volunteers received a 250 ml infusion of stroma-free haemoglobin at a rate of 2–4 ml/min. The haemoglobin concentration of this solution was 6.4 g/dl. The P_{50} was not reported. Two control patients received similar infusions of 5% albumin.

The most striking finding of this study was a decline in creatinine clearance in the haemoglobin solution recipients from a baseline value of

148 ml/min to 73 ml/min 1 hour after infusion. This value returned to normal in the second hour following infusion. This alteration in kidney function was accompanied by a sharp decline in urine volume in these patients. In the albumin control patients no changes were seen in urine volume or creatinine clearance. The authors stressed that this deterioration in kidney function was transient and not associated with permanent renal damage. Nevertheless, these results had a chilling effect on further clinical research.

As Savitsky et al pointed out, there are three possible explanations for the observed nephrotoxicity. The first is stromal toxicity. They did report a stroma lipid level of 1.6 mg/dl. Since this represents only 1% of the original level of phospholipid, and since the infusion of haemoglobin solution did not produce detectable disseminated intravascular coagulation in the recipients, stromal toxicity is an unlikely explanation. A second possibility is the presence of a vasoactive substance in the haemoglobin solution that affects renal blood flow. This is supported by the observation that seven of the eight haemoglobin recipients developed transient bradycardia and mild hypertension during the infusion. We noted similar findings in our early heamoglobin solution studies in baboons. We therefore believe that prospective haemoglobin solutions should be tested for the presence of vasoactive substances by bioassay techniques prior to clinical testing.

A third possibility is that the changes in renal function were simply related to the filtration of free haemoglobin through the kidneys. Perhaps haemoglobin filtration in some way interferes with normal kidney function. Once the haemoglobinemia disappears, renal function returns to normal. This is an interesting argument, since the highest level of plasma haemoglobin in the human volunteers was only 57 mg/dl. In actual clinical practice, we expect plasma haemoglobin levels to rise to 6 to 8 gm/dl, a thousandfold increase over the levels seen in the clinical safety trials. It is likely that elevations of plasma haemoglobin of that magnitude would produce even greater changes in renal function, especially in a setting of haemorrhagic shock.

It should be emphasized that the pyrogen free haemoglobin solution used by Savitsky et al in the most recent clinical trial, was tested for renal effects in both dogs and monkeys. None of the effects seen in the human volunteers was observed in the animal studies. Renal dysfunction has been the primary source of concern with respect to the clinical use of haemoglobin solution. The absence of a dependable animal model that would mimic the clinical findings, has thus been a major hurdle to any future clinical trials.

We have recently reported on a well hydrated unanesthetized baboon model for the study of renal function (Moss et al 1986, Rosen et al 1986b). This model reproducibly shows the haemodynamic and renal effects that were reported by Savitsky et al with the infusion of SFH while showing no changes with the infusion of Ringer's lactate solution. These findings are shown in Table 8.5. It is possible that in this model the adverse

Table 8.5   Haemodynamic and renal response to unmodified stroma-free haemoglobin (SFH).

	Baseline	Post-Infusion of SFH
Heart Rate (bpm)	114 ± 9	90 ± 7*
MAP (torr)	114 ± 4	133 ± 3*
Urine output (ml)	201 ± 48	91 ± 22*
GFR (ml/min/m²)	87.9 ± 7.5	67.2 ± 5.8*

* Changes significant (p < 0.025)

haemodynamic and renal effects will not be seen with poly SFH-P, since it does not clear the kidneys. The availability of this model will now permit a proper evaluation of all haemoglobin based red cell substitutes for adverse haemodynamic and renal effects. This will eliminate a major hurdle in pre-clinical investigations of haemoglobin solutions.

Our second concern is postinfusion immunosuppression. Since sepsis is one of the most serious complications that might develop in circumstances where haemoglobin solution would be used, it is important to establish that the infusion of haemoglobin solution will not impair the host defense mechanism.

The effect of haemoglobin solution on granulocyte function was evaluated (Hau et al 1980). It was shown that haemoglobin acted as an adjuvant in experimental peritonitis in rats by interfering with granulocyte phagocytosis and bacterial killing capability. However, the significance of this finding is not clear, since the haemoglobin only acted as an adjuvant when it was injected into the peritoneal cavity. It was not effective when it was injected intravenously or intramuscularly. In another report, Hoyt et al (1981) studied the ability of rats to withstand peritonitis following exposure to haemoglobin solution used as a volume expander in the treatment of haemorrhagic shock. They found no evidence that haemoglobin solution depressed host defense mechanisms.

Whether poly SFH-P alters immunocompetence is unknown. It is known that the infusion of colloid particles produces blockade of the reticulo-endothelial system and thereby enhances susceptibility to bacterial toxins (Litwin et al 1963). It has been demonstrated that the infusion of colloid particles not only blocks the reticuloendothelial system but also produces an acute depletion of plasma fibronectin levels (Stein et al 1979). Thus studies designed to investigate the effects of poly SFH-P on immunocompetence would be necessary prior to clinical trials.

LIPID ENCAPSULATED HAEMOGLOBIN

An alternate approach for a haemoglobin based red cell substitute is one that encapsulates the haemoglobin in an artificial membrane (haemosomes). Unmodified stroma-free haemoglobin can be readily encapsulated in a lipid membrane, consisting of a mixture of phospholipids and cholesterol (Djordjevich et al 1980).

Even though the concept of haemoglobin and the enzymic contents of red cells encapsulated in an artificial membrane is probably the most attractive, efforts at proving its efficacy are in their infancy. A few studies report on the survival of rats following a 90% exchange with haemosomes (Hunt et al 1985, Mayoral et al 1985). Proof of its efficacy would have been more conclusive if the investigators had carried out a complete washout of the red cells to a haematocrit of O. This is particularly true since the methodology to assess the efficacy of O_2 transport of haemosomes in the presence of red cells has not yet been developed. Results of these early studies are encouraging, however, and need to be pursued.

One problem that has plagued haemosome research has been the inability to prepare a reproducible haemosomal suspension in litre quantities and have a particle size distribution such that sterilizing through a 0.22 μ filter would be feasible. Some progress has been made in this regard by use of a Microfluidizer (Farmer et al 1985). However, all current haemosomal preparations have approximately half the normal oxygen carrying capacity, but can be readily made to have a normal P_{50}.

Encapsulation of haemoglobin has not resulted in a consistent increase in the intravascular half-life compared to the unmodified tetramer. Depending on the preparations technique, the $T_{1/2}$ varies from 6 hours to 15 hours compared with 2–4 hours for the unmodified SFH. A smaller particle size distribution appears to improve the $T_{1/2}$.

The potential toxicity of haemosomes has not been investigated to any significant extent. Though several preliminary studies do not suggest any acute toxicity (Hunt et al 1985), long term effects of haemosomes have not been addressed. This approach still remains a very attractive one, and hopefully greater effort will be put in this direction.

In summary, a review of the literature suggests that, since the first report on poly SFH-P, many investigators view it as the most likely candidate solution that could circumvent all the major problems that have precluded the clinical use of haemoglobin based red cell substitutes. The outcome of the ongoing investigations on issues of safety will ultimately determine the clinical use of poly SFH-P.

REFERENCES

Amberson W R 1934 Blood substitutes. Biological Reviews of the Cambridge Philosophical Society 12: 48–86

Amberson W R, Flexner J, Steggerda F R et al 1934 On the use of Ringer-Locke solutions containing hemoglobin as a substitute for normal blood in mammals. Journal of Cellular Comparrative Physiology 5: 359–382

Amberson W R, Jennings J J, Rhode C M 1949 Clinical experience with hemoglobin-saline solutions. Journal of Applied Physiology 1: 469–489

Ajisaka K, Iwashita Y 1980 Modification of human hemoglobin with polyethylene glycol: A new candidate for blood substitute. Biochemical and Biophysical Research Communications 97: 1076–1081

Baldwin J E, Gill B, Whitten J P 1981 Synthesis of polymer-bound hemoglobin samples. Tetrahedion 37: 1723–1726

Benesch R E, Benesch R, Renthal R D 1972 Affinity labelling of the polyphosphate binding site of hemoglobin. Biochemistry 11: 3576–3582

Benesch R E, Yung S, Suzuki T, Bauer C, Benesch R 1975 Pyridoxal compounds as specific reagents for the alpha and beta N-terminal of hemoglobin. Proceedings of National Academy of Science USA 70: 2595–2599

Birndorf N I, Lopas H L 1970 Effect of red cell stroma-free hemoglobin solution on renal function in monkeys. Journal of Applied Physiology 29: 573–577

Birndorf N I, Lopas H L, Robbay S 1971 Disseminated intravascular coagulation and renal failures. Laboratory Investigation 25:314

Blumenstein J, Tain S C, Chang J E, Wong J T 1978 Experimental transfusion of dextran-hemoglobin. Progress in Clinical and Biological Research 19: 205–212

Board P G, Pidcock M E 1981 Methaemoglobinaemia Resulting from heterozygosity for two NADH-methaemoglobin reductase variants: Characterization as NADH-ferricyanide reductase. British Journal of Haematology 47: 361–370

Bonsen P, Laver M B, Morris K C 1977 Blood substitute and plasma expander comprising polyhemoglobin. US Patent 4 0001 401

Cannan R K, Redish J 1942 The large scale production of crystalline human hemoglobin with preliminary observations on the effect of its injection in man. In: Blood substitutes and blood transfusions. S Mudd and W Thalhimer (eds) Charles C Thomas, Springfield, IL, p 147–155

DeVenuto F, Zuck T F, Zegna A I, Moores W Y 1977 Characteristics of stroma-free hemoglobin prepared by crystallization. Journal of Laboratory Clinical Medicine 80: 509–516

DeVenuto F, Zegna A I 1981 Transfusion with pyridoxylated-polymerized hemoglobin solution. Transfusion 21:599

DeVenuto F, Zegna A I 1982 Blood Exchange with pyridoxylated and polymerized hemoglobin solution. Surgery Gynaecology and obstetrics 155: 342–246

Djordjevich L, Millier I F 1980 Synthetic erythrocytes from lipid encapsulated hemoglobin. Experimental Hematology 584–592

Dodge J T, Mitchell C, Hanahan D J 1963 The preparation and chemical characteristics of hemoglobin free ghosts of human erythrocytes. Archives of Biochemistry and Biophysics 100: 119–130

Farmer M C, Beissinger R L, Gossage J L 1985 Liposome encapsulated hemoglobin as a red cell surrogate. ACEMB

Feola M, Gonzalez H, Canizaro P C 1983 Development of a bovine stroma-free hemoglobin solution as a blood substitute. 157: 399–408

Gould S A, Rosen A L, Sehgal L R et al 1980 The effect of altered hemoglobin-oxygen affinity on oxygen transport by stroma-free hemoglobin. Journal of Surgical Research

Gould S A, Sehgal L R, Rosen A L et al 1982 Hemoglobin solution: Is a normal [Hb] or P_{50} more important? Journal of Surgical Research 33: 189–193

Gould S A, Sehgal L R, Rosen A L, Sehgal H L, Moss G S 1985 Polyhemoglobin: An improved red blood cell substitute. Surgical Forum 36: 30–31

Gould S A, Rosen A L, Sehgal L R, Sehgal H L, Moss G S, 1986 Polymerized pyridoxylated hemoglobin: Efficacy as an O_2 carrier. Journal of Trauma (in press)

Greenburg A G, Schooley M, Peskin G W 1977 Improved retention of stroma-free hemoglobin solution by chemical modification. Journal of Trauma 17: 501–504

Hamilton P B, Farr L e, Hiller A 1947 Preparation of hemoglobin solutions for intravenous infusion. Journal of Experimental Medicine 86:455

Hau T, Simmons R L 1980 Mechanism of the adjuvant effect of hemoglobin on phagocytosis and intracellular killing by human granulocytes. Surgery 87: 588–592

Horowitz B, Mazur A 1978 Oxygen equilibrium and structure studies of amidinated human hemoglobin. Progress in Clinical and Biological Research 19: 149–165

Hoyt D B, Greenburg A G, Peskin G W, Forbes S, Reese H 1981 Resuscitation with pyridoxylated stroma-free hemoglobin: Tolerance of sepsis. Journal of Trauma 21: 938–942

Hunt C A, Burnette R R, MacGregor R D, Strubbe A E 1985 Synthesis and evaluation of a prototypal artificial red cell. Science 1165–1168

Kiepert P E, Chang T M S 1984 Preparation and in vitro characteristics of a blood substitute based on pyridoxylated polyhemoglobin. Applied Biochemistry and Biotechnology 10: 133–141

Kiepert P E, Chang T M S 1985 Pyridoxylated polyhemoglobin as a red cell substitute for resuscitation of lethal hemorrhagic shock in conscious rats. Biomaterials, Medical Devices and Artificial Organs 13: 1–15

Kothe N, Eichentopf B, Bonhard K 1985 Characterization of modified, stroma-free hemoglobin solution as an oxygen-carrying plasma substitute Surgical Obstetrics and gynaecology 161: 563–569

Litwin M D, Walter C W, Ejarqne P, Reynolds E S 1963 Synergistic toxicity of gram negative bacteria and free colloidal hemoglobin. Annals of Surgery 157: 485–493

Mayoral J, Djordjevich L, Miller I F, Ivankovich, A D 1985 Evaluation of synthetic erythrocytes as blood substitutes. ACEMB

Mok W, Chen D, Mazur A 1975 Cross-linked hemoglobin as potential plasma protein extenders. Federation Proceedings 34: 1458–1460

Morris K C, Bonsen P, Laver M B 1977 Pharmaceutically acceptable intramolecularly cross-linked stroma-free hemoglobin. US Patent 4 061 736

Moss G S, DeWoskin R, Cochin A 1973 Stroma-free hemoglobin. Preparation and observations on in vitro changes in coagulation. Surgery 74:198

Moss G S, DeWoskin R, Rosen A L, Levine H, Palani C K 1976 Transport of oxygen and carbon dioxide by hemoglobin-saline solution in the red cell free primate. Surgery, Gynecology and Obstetrics 142: 357–362

Moss G S, Gould S A, Rosen A L, Sehgal L R, Sehgal H L 1986 Animal model for nephrotoxicity of hemoglobin tetramer. Lancet 1:1219

Mulder A G, Amberson W R, Steggerda F R, Flexner J 1934 Oxygen consumption with hemoglobin ringer. Journal of Cellular Comparative Physiology 5: 383–397

Rabiner S F, Helbert J R, Lopas H, Friedman L H 1967 Evaluation of a stroma-free hemoglobin solution for use as a plasma expander. Journal of Experimental Medicine 126: 1127–1142

Rabiner S F, Friedman L H 1968 The role of intravascular hemolysis and the reticuloendothelial system in the production of a hypercoagulable slate. British Journal of Haematology 14: 105–118

Riggs T E, Shafer A W, Guenter C A 1973 Acute changes oxyhemoglobin affinity. Journal of Clinical Investigation 52:2660

Rosen A L, Gould S A, Sehgal L R, Sehgal H L, Moss G S 1983 Evaluation of efficacy of stroma-free hemoglobin solutions. In: Bolin R B, Geyer R P, Nemo G J (eds) Advances in blood substitute research Alan R. Liss, New York 59–70

Rosen A L, Sehgal L R, Gould S A, Sehgal H L, Moss G S 1986a Methodology to assess the oxygen concentration of red cells and stroma-free hemoglobin solutions. Critical Care Medicine 14: 147–150

Rosen A L, Sehgal L R, Gould S A, Sehgal H L, DeWoskin R, Moss G S 1986b Renal response to hemoglobin solutions. Physiologist 29: 532

Rozenburg G Y 1978 Chemically modified hemoglobin. An artificial oxygen transporter. Doklady Academii Nauk SSSR 243: 1320–1323

Savitsky J P, Doczi J, Black J, Arnold J D 1978 A clinical safety trial of stroma-free hemoglobin. Clinical Pharmacology and Therapeutics 23: 73–80

Sehgal L R, Rosen A L, Gould S A et al 1980 In vitro and in vivo characteristics of polymerized pyridoxylated hemoglobin solution. Federation Proceedings 39:2383

Sehgal L R, Rosen A L, Noud G et al 1981 Large volume preparation of pyridoxylated hemoglobin with high P_{50}. Journal of Surgical Research 30: 14–20

Sehgal L R, Rosen A L, Gould S A, Sehgal H L, Moss G S 1983a An appraisal of polymerized pyridoxylated hemoglobin as an acellular oxygen carrier. In: Bolin R B, Geyer R P, Nemo G J (eds) Advances in blood substitute research. Alan R. Liss, New York 19–28

Sehgal L R, Rosen A L, Gould S A, Sehgal H L, Moss G S 1983b Preparation and in vitro characteristics of polymerized pyridoxylated hemoglobin. Transfusion 23: 158–162

Sehgal L R, Gould S A, Rosen A L, Sehgal H L, Moss G S 1984 Polymerized pyridoxylated hemoglobin: A red cell substitute with normal oxygen capacity. Surgery 95: 433–438

Sellards A W, Minot G R 1916 Injection of hemoglobin in man and its relation to blood destruction, with especial reference to the anemia. Journal of Medical Research 34: 469–494

Stein P M, Saba T M 1979 Cardiovascular response to hemorrhage in the dog as modified by colloid induced opsonic deficiency and reticuloendothelial blockade. Federation Proceedings 38:1115

Cost-containment in transfusion practice: A view from the United States

INTRODUCTION

The unremitting escalation of medical care costs over the past two decades has finally met with resistance. While this issue was addressed in the United Kingdom years ago, only recently has legislation been enacted in the United States to curb such expenses. Sweeping reforms in the health care reimbursement system promise to usher in the most sudden and dramatic changes in health care delivery seen during the past half-century.

Before 1983, medical services in the United States were reimbursed retrospectively on the basis of charges for services provided. Both hospital and physician fees were covered in this manner. Vested interests hindered motivation to control costs. Under the new system (Tax Equity and Fiscal Responsibility Act 1982, Social Security Amendments, Public Law 98–21: 1983), reimbursement for health care services covered by federal programmes is prospective and based upon 'reasonable' costs for delivery of services. A schedule of fees for hospital services deemed appropriate for various illnesses and procedures is assigned on the basis of diagnosis-related groupings. Institutions which treat patients within preset guidelines profit, while those which exceed the guidelines obviously suffer. Currently, the programme applies only to services provided for the elderly, the poor and the chronically ill; however, it is anticipated that private health insurance carriers will follow the Government's lead.

The following discussion will assess the issues involved under the new system with relation to blood transfusion services and will outline approaches to deal with this new era in health care delivery.

ADMINISTRATIVE CONCERNS

The new reimbursement system has had a profound impact on clinical laboratories. Efforts by administrators to reduce operational costs are hampered by the fact that the laboratories respond to requests for tests from clinicians and cannot directly reduce their work volume. Moreover, for some clinical laboratories, as well as other health care support areas such as radiology, excessive ordering of tests is a defensive practice related to malpractice litigation. Nevertheless, there is a need to maximize laboratory productivity for clinically relevant work and the blood bank community has, perhaps more than workers in other disciplines, responded to this challenge. This has resulted in careful scrutiny of the need for tests to be performed and has occasioned efforts to ensure maximization of efficiency with regard to technologist workload and maximization of relevance with regard to clinical applications of specific tests.

The new system has also changed the way in which health support areas are viewed by hospital administrators. Although the laboratories are not the major source of hospital costs, they represent a highly visible target since they are now a 'cost centre' for the institution rather than a 'profit-centre'.

In considering the costs of laboratory services to a hospital, one must presently consider space requirements, personnel, expenses for commodities, capital equipment and waste. Excessive space assignment deprives the hospital from use of that space for revenue-producing activities. Moreover, the overhead for maintenance increases the hospital's cost without the potential of realizing offsetting revenue. Personnel expense, however, is the most significant concern. It has become important to balance personnel assignments in the various hospital laboratories as well as to ensure equity of staffing between shifts as related to work volume. This is facilitated by use of workload statistics (College of American Pathologists 1984). Further, duplication of effort by laboratories is extremely costly; therefore, efforts toward consolidation and centralization of laboratory functions are appropriate.

Commodity expenses are difficult to control unless there is modification of laboratory procedures or a decrease in demand for services. In the blood bank, the most expensive commodity is blood and its components, and reducing utilization through education of medical staff is most important, although very difficuit to achieve. Elimination of unnecessary testing also will reduce commodity expenses but this usually has only a minor impact. Capital equipment expenditure in blood banks is minimal in comparison with other clinical laboratories. Also, the era of cost containment has resulted in a reluctance to purchase expensive equipment unless such equipment can generate revenue for the institution, or lead to more efficient laboratory testing with a concomitant reduction in personnel. Finally, avoidance of waste, particularly of commodities, is extremely important. In the blood bank, such wastage primarily involves outdating of whole blood, blood components and reagents. Control of inventory through such concepts as surgical blood order schedules or inventory rotation between institutions are useful practices. In instances where recalcitrance on the part of medical staff makes control of outdating difficult, marketing of outdated blood for research or fractionation may prove feasible.

While there is concern for control of laboratory costs, there is equal concern for realization of new sources of revenue which can offset expenditure by the clinical laboratories. New patient care programmes provided by blood banks, especially those in larger hospitals, such as therapeutic plasma exchange, outpatient transfusion, testing for HLA and platelet antigens, reference laboratory antibody identification studies and paternity testing, may result in additional revenue.

BLOOD PROCUREMENT ACTIVITIES

The practice of each hospital having its own blood collection facility waned during the past decade for economic reasons. Although an on-site collection facility is a convenience, particularly for a large hospital, it is an extremely expensive one. The cost of recruitment of new blood donors, as well as the cost of space and of additional laboratory personel, preclude such operations. In contrast, centralization of blood collection within a community results in much more efficient use of personnel and enhances efficient use of the blood supply. Further, centralization of donor recruitment not only is cost-effective, but also avoids potential confusion in the minds of the public when they are confronted with requests from a variety of donor collection programmes.

Centralization of blood procurement is usually linked to centralized testing of collected blood. In addition, community programmes often provide reference laboratory support and, in some instances, perform pretransfusion tests on prospective recipients. This can further reduce personnel and space requirements for blood bank services in area hospitals. Moreover, the larger volume and more predictable testing schedules which result from centralization allows the regional facility to purchase automated equipment which further conserves personnel expenses.

There is concern that centralized testing may result in a monopoly with the inherent potential for inflated charges. While this is a distinct possibility, it can be avoided by inclusion of consumers (e.g. hospital blood bank directors) on the governing board of the centralized facility. Yet another concern is that competition among blood providers, although possibly resulting in lower costs for blood and blood components, would have a negative impact on orderly donor recruitment.

For the hospital, centralization assumes considerable importance in terms of cost containment since it allows for alternative space utilization. Rather than providing hospital space for intermittent collection of blood, and staffing of that area with secretarial, recruitment and technical or nursing staff, the space and personnel can be assigned to revenue-producing activities such as outpatient transfusion and therapeutic plasma exchange. Both of these services are better performed in a hospital than in a centralized collection facility since expert medical care is more likely to be readily available. In addition, provision of these services in a hospital, rather than in a centralized community blood bank, is convenient for patients in that they can be treated in proximity to their attending physician. Activities which lend themselves to prior scheduling, and thereby avoid disruption of staffing patterns, are also feasible in this setting. For example, collection of autologous blood for transfusion during subsequent operations is better performed in a hospital than in a centralized facility.

An important factor in determining the feasibility of centralization of blood resources is the efficiency of blood delivery. Centralization should be reconsidered if the charges for supply of blood and blood components by a centralized facility exceed the total cost of these functions performed by a hospital. It is important to include such often-overlooked factors as the cost of space in the hospital and the potential use of that space for alternative revenue production. Centralization also must be reconsidered if the centralized facility's inability to meet a hospital's needs for blood results in frequent cancellation or postponement of operative procedures. In the latter instance, some degree of competition may benefit the over-all situation. However, mere redirection of the community blood donor pool without an increase in the number of donors is not a solution. In such a situation, an additional centralized facility using more effective donor recruitment would be preferable to returning to a system of donor rooms in each hospital.

Hospital size, location and pattern of medical care also influences the feasibility of blood collection by hospitals. For example, a solitary tertiary care institution which requires such components as granulocytes and HLA matched platelets, may well find that a centralized blood bank does not find it economical to provide such products when no other hospital in the area requires them. In this instance the tertiary care institution may elect to maintain its own donor room.

A final factor related to blood collection is the current enthusiasm for donors to provide blood for friends and family members. The impetus for this relates to the fear of transmission of infections diseases, especially hepatitis and acquired immune deficiency syndrome. The medical community generally agrees that such directed donation is unnecessary. However, those hospitals which maintain blood collection facilities have a more difficult time withstanding pressures for such requests than do hospitals which lack them.

SEROLOGICAL TESTING

In the current economic environment it is prudent, if not essential, to eliminate tests unless the data obtained influence transfusion management or aid in patient diagnosis. For example, testing prospective recipient bloods with anti-A, B originally was undertaken to recognize inactive anti-A or anti-B, or the omission of either reagent from test tubes. With the use of color-coded antisera and quality assurance programmes these reasons are no longer valid. While it can be argued that use of anti-A, B provides a means of detecting ABO subgroups, such as A_x, group O blood is generally transfused to A_x recipients. In routine practice the use of anti-A, B is best reserved for confirming the ABO type of units labelled as group O. Similarly, ascertaining the D^u status of a patient's red cells which type as D-negative by direct agglutination tests is redundant; Rh-negative blood can be administered regardless of the D^u test results. D^u testing can be limited to those apparent D-negative transfusion candidates requiring large volumes of blood; Rh-positive blood can be administered to those found to be D^u.

A further consideration is the need for testing beyond that mandated by accrediting agencies. Only if such studies are proven cost-effective can they be justified. The cost-effectiveness of any laboratory test is not easily determined. It is relatively simple to project direct cost-savings related to costs for reagents and other supplies, but a larger benefit will be realized if personnel expenses can be reduced. Personnel costs/test can be determined using the Workload Recording Method devised by the College of American Pathologists (Perryman 1982).

New technology may permit streamlining of existing test protocols and realize modest cost-savings. This is seen with use of chemically modified anti-D reagents which contain reduced and alkylated IgG molecules prepared in a low-protein diluent. Unlike reagents prepared in a high-protein diluent, chemically modified antisera are not prone to yield false-positive results with red blood cells (RBCs) from patients with autoimmune disease states (Widmann 1985). A separate, concurrent, Rh control test is required to detect such false-positive results when high-protein reagents are used. However, with chemically modified antisera, negative reactions with either anti-A or -B, having a protein content similar to that of the chemically modified anti-D, obviate the need for an additional control test on all samples except those from group AB patients. Also, use of monoclonal antisera for ABO typing avoids detection of ABO anomalies that are often of academic interest, such as the acquired-B phenomenon and RBC poly-agglutination. Further, whereas A subgroups usually react weakly with human source antisera they generally react strongly with monoclonal anti-A. Thus, the need for additional studies to resolve such problems is greatly reduced. Other developments that may reduce costs include use of micro-plate and solid-phase techniques, and automation.

In some instances additional savings can be realized if the specificity of a procedure can be improved, thereby reducing the number of false-positive tests which necessitate time-consuming and costly resolution, and thereby may prolong hospitalization. The latter is an overriding concern in any cost containment programme. However, patient safety must not be compromised by reducing sensitivity of methods, since this can result in an extension of hospital stay. Moreover, the costs of successful litigation resulting from inappropriate practices will far exceed any cost-savings attained through streamlining serological testing. It is essential, therefore, to ensure that test protocols conform to regionally accepted standards.

Table 9.1   Required serological testing.

Donor bloods

ABO — RBCs with anti-A and anti-B; serum/plasma with A_1 and B RBCs
— confirmatory testing by transfusing facility

Rh — anti-D; D^u test on apparent D-negatives
— confirmatory D^u test on D-negatives by transfusing facility

antibody — methods that demonstrate clinically significant antibodies active at
detection   37°C, but only donors with a prior history of transfusion or
pregnancy

HBsAg — method not specified

syphilis — method not specified (FDA requirement only)

anti-HIV — Western blots on repeat ELISA positives

Recipient bloods

ABO — RBCs with anti-A and anti-B; serum/plasma with A_1 and B RBCs

Rh — anti-D by direct agglutination and a control test for autoagglutination

antibody — methods that demonstrate clinically significant antibodies active at
detection   37°c including an antiglobulin test with RBCs that are not pooled
— control test for false-negatives

crossmatch — test for ABO incompatibility except if unexpected antibodies are, or
are known to have been, present; if so, antiglobulin crossmatch
required

Prenatal patients

Rh — anti-D; D^u test on apparent D-negatives including a method to detect
false-positives due to a large fetal-maternal hemorrhage (FMH)

antibody — for anti-D on D-negatives
detection

FMH screen — a test to detect FMH in excess of 15 ml RBCs

The required extent of serological practice in the United States is governed principally by the Standards for Blood Banks and Transfusion Services (Holland & Schmidt 1987) and, to a lesser extent, by the Code of Federal Regulations (Office of Biologics 1984) and the Commission on Laboratory Accreditation (College of American Pathologists 1985). Tests currently required are summarized in Table 9.1. While these are considered minimum performance requirements, acceptable procedures are often not stipulated. For example, unexpected antibodies must be detected by methods that demonstrate clinically significant antibodies, including 37°C incubation and an antiglobulin test. 'Clinically significant' is undefined and the antigen profile of the RBCs, suitable test media, minimum incubation times, criteria for antiglobulin sera and the need for microscopic examination of serological tests, are not specified.

In the ensuing discussion, technical considerations which affect personnel conservation and/or commodity costs will be addressed in relation to three procedures: screening tests for unexpected antibodies, the direct antiglobulin test (autocontrol) and the crossmatch.

Screening tests for unexpected antibodies

Screening sera from prospective transfusion recipients for unexpected antibodies is a required component of compatibility testing in the United

States. Such testing should be undertaken sufficiently in advance of the crossmatch to allow for early recognition of problem cases. This facilitates such inventory management practices as 'Type and Screen' (T & S) (Boral & Henry 1977) and Maximum Surgical Blood Ordering Schedules (MSBOS) (Friedman et al 1976).

What constitutes an adequate screening protocol? While mandating 37°C incubation and use of the antiglobulin technique, the Standards for Blood Banks and Transfusion Services (Holland & Schmidt 1987) preclude use of pooled reagent RBCs and require performance of a test to detect false-negative results. The latter entails addition of IgG-coated RBCs to nonreactive antiglobulin tests. Both changes were introduced in conjunction with relaxation of prerequisites for donor-recipient compatibility testing; namely, the antiglobulin phase of the crossmatch may be omitted providing no clinically significant unexpected antibodies are detected in screening tests, and there is no prior history of such antibodies.

In spite of these requirements, a wide array of methods may be utilized, including saline, albumin, low-ionic-strength saline (LISS), Polybrene^R and enzyme techniques. Sera may be tested against two or more reagent RBC samples. Tests may be incubated at room temperature (RT) and 37°C, or only at 37°C. The antihuman globulin (AHG) phase may be performed with anti-IgG or with a polyspecific reagent containing anti-IgG and anticomplement (anti-C3). Tests may be examined macroscopically, with or without an optical aid, or viewed microscopically. Coupled with variations in incubation times and serum to red cell ratios the procedural permutations seem infinite. Let us examine the issues involved in selecting a procedure for pretransfusion antibody detection.

Serological technique

Speed, sensitivity, specificity and simplicity are fundamental considerations in the selection of an appropriate antibody screening protocol; all have an impact on operational costs. Among the various methods available, an albumin test read after incubation at 37°C with subsequent testing by the indirect antiglobulin technique (IAT) is widely employed. Such a technique detects most clinically significant antibodies and is not associated with an inordinate number of unwanted positive tests. LISS techniques, which allow for reduction of incubation times, are also popular. Data indicating the relative sensitivity and specificity of both methods are shown in Table 9.2. With the realization that *no* currently available method will detect *all* clinically significant antibodies, our laboratory utilizes a LISS-wash procedure, incubating serum with two reagent RBC samples for 10 minutes at 37°C without a RT phase, followed by washing before the antiglobulin reaction with polyspecific AHG and viewing reactions with the aid of an illuminated concave mirror. Such a protocol is associated with a unwanted positive rate of 0.61% and fails to detect one potentially clinically significant antibody among approximately 5000 samples (Table 9.3).

Table 9.2 Role of albumin, LISS, polyspecific AHG and anti-IgG in the detection of unexpected antibodies. (After Garratty 1985.)

Method	Antibodies missed	% Unwanted positives
RT-37-LISS-PS	0	1.41
37-LISS-PS	0	0.61
RT-37-ALB-PS	6	0.21
37-ALB-PS	6	0.1
37-LISS-IG	5	0.1
37-ALB-IG	10	0.1

Table 9.3 Unexpected antibodies detected by crossmatch but not in screening tests* with reagent red cells[†].

Antibody specificities	Clinical significance
$-C$; $-c$; $-C^w$; $-E$ (5)	potentially
$-Fy^a$; $-Fy^b$; $-Jk^a$ (2)	significant
$-Js^a$; $-K$ (2); $-V$; $-Wr^a$	(n = 17)
$-A_1Le^{bH}$; $-Bg$ (5); $-Le^a$ (4)	doubtful
$-Le^a+M$; $-Le^a+P_1$; $-Le^b$ (2)	significance
$-Lu^a$ (7); $-M$ (9); $-P_1$ (7)	(n = 37)
miscellaneous (auto-I/HI, etc.)	insignificant
	(n = 77)

* Tests on 81 444 prospective recipient blood samples, University of Michigan data, 1983–1984
[†] R_1R_1 and R_2R_2 phenotypes used in LISS tests at 37°C and by the indirect antiglobulin technique

Reagent red cells

Commercially available R_1R_1 and R_2R_2 reagent RBCs are, with few limitations, adequate for routine antibody detection. Preferably both samples should be devoid of Bg antigens. Failure by the manufacturer to meet this requirement can account for positive reactions with approximately 1% of pretransfusion samples, resulting in time-consuming and costly investigations which may prolong patient care.

The need for more than two reagent RBC samples to ensure detection of dosing antibodies and antibodies to low-incidence antigens must be questioned. Our failure to detect the 17 potentially clinically significantly alloantibodies listed in Table 9.2 was related to dosage in only two instances (one anti-Fy^a and one anti-Jk^a). (Dosage is also discussed below with regard to the recognition of those Kidd-system antibodies that are nonreactive in tests with anti-IgG.) Moreover, it is difficult to conceive that any practical increase in the number of reagent RBC samples would have ensured detection of the four antibodies to low-incidence antigens (anti-C^w, -V, -Js^a and -Wr^a).

Each additional reagent RBC sample used in the procedure results in a 50% increase in direct costs. In our opinion, such increased testing to facilitate detection of rare, weakly-reactive, albeit potentially significant, antibodies cannot be justified.

Room temperature incubation

With the realization that alloantibodies reactive only below 37°C do not cause significant RBC destruction (Mollison 1983, Issitt 1985), many investigators abandoned RT tests except for an immediate-spin (IS) crossmatch to recognize ABO incompatibility. However, some cold-reactive antibodies react even in IS tests. Delay in patient care and workload related to problem solving are greatly reduced by using LISS tests at 37°C without an IS phase. This permits recognition of ABO errors yet avoids detection of IS-reactive antibodies of no clinical significance (Trudeau et al 1983).

Incubation times

Using LISS rather than albumin reduces incubation times, and thereby accelerates the availability of blood for transfusion. This enhances the acceptance of preoperative blood order schedules by surgeons. However, while relative incubation times need to be considered, the amount of 'hands-on' time involved is of paramount importance. Thus, the LISS-wash procedure (Moore & Mollison 1976) has not been adopted as widely as LISS-additive methods. Moreover, while the manual Polybrene® test (Lalezari & Jiang 1980) entails only a one minute incubation, it is not popularly utilized because of the required expertise and 'hands-on' time.

Microscopic examination of tests

Routine use of the microscope in the blood bank creates far more problems than it solves (Issitt 1985). Of particular concern is the increased number of unwanted positive reactions due to clinically insignificant antibodies (e.g. autoanti-I, -HI) that entail fruitless evaluation and needless patient care delay. Nonetheless, it is likely that some of the antibodies listed in Table 9.3 would have been detected by microscopic reading of tests.

Enzyme tests

Inclusion of enzyme tests in pretransfusion studies affords detection of 'enzyme-only' antibodies, some of which have Rh-related specificity of questionable clinical significance (Issitt 1979). However, use of enzyme tests does not reduce the incidence of delayed haemolytic transfusion reactions and therefore cannot be considered cost-effective (Riglin & Patten 1985). Moreover, while we have no data comparing the sensitivity of LISS-IAT with enzyme-IAT, we have yet, after four years of retrospective study, to observe an 'enzyme-only' alloantibody that was responsible for a delayed haemolytic transfusion reaction. In the light of this, coupled with the associated increased direct costs, we do not use enzyme tests for routine antibody detection.

Anti-C3 in AHG

The need for anti-C3 activity in AHG has been the subject of considerable debate in the past decade, originating with a letter to the Editor of Transfusion which concluded that effective alloantibody detection is not dependent upon the anti-C3 activity of AHG (Beck & Marsh 1977). Unfortunately no supporting data were presented. This prompted others to undertake definitive studies. It was shown that some alloantibodies with specificities in the Duffy, Kell, Kidd, SsU, Cartwright and Colton systems react at a higher dilution in tests with polyspecific AHG than in tests with anti-IgG alone (Wright & Issitt 1979). In another study, the anti-C3 activity in polyspecific AHG was essential for the detection of eight potentially clinically significant alloantibodies (six anti-Jk^a, one anti-Jk^b and one one antibody to a low-incidence antigen) in 38 854 sera (Howard et al 1982). The seven Kidd-system antibodies represented 23% of all anti-Jk^a/-Jk^b found. However, use of polyspecific AHG results in the detection of unwanted positive tests associated with clinically insignificant C3-binding antibodies (Garratty 1985). When LISS-IATs are performed the incidence of such unwanted positive test is 0.61%. This figure can be reduced to 0.1% by performing LISS-IATs with anti-IgG (Table 9.2).

Dosage considerations

It has been recommended recently that a double dose expression of Jk^a be present on reagent RBCs used in pretransfusion screening tests for unexpected serum antibodies (Shulman et al 1985). This recommendation was based on data from albumin tests with anti-IgG. Twelve of 26 anti-Jk^a detected among 169 791 samples failed to react with Jk(a+b+) RBCs. No recommendations were made regarding the detection of anti-Jk^b.

Our own data confirm and extend these observations. In tests on 37 of 60 Kidd-system antibodies (28 anti-Jk^a and 9 anti-Jk^b) detected with polyspecific AHG in LISS-IATs employed as part of 56 514 screening tests for unexpected antibodies, we found that dosage, use of polyspecific AHG or proteases, and increasing incubation times, all enhanced detection of these antibodies. Moreover, 14 of the 37 antibodies tested (10 anti-Jk^a, 4 anti-Jk^b) were not reactive with anti-IgG in tests against Jk(a+b+) RBCs; eight failed

Table 9.4 Influence of incubation time, polyspecific AHG and dosage on the detection of Kidd-system antibodies by LISS-IAT[†].

Incubation time	Antiglobulin serum	Dosage + + +	
10′	polyspecific	37[*]	29
15′	polyspecific	37	33
10′	anti-IgG	34	23

[*] Number of Kidd-system antibodies detected
[†] University of Michigan data, 1984–1985

to react with Jk(a+b+) red cells when polyspecific AHG was used in 10-minute LISS tests but four were detected in 15-minute tests, and three antibodies were nonreactive in tests with anti-IgG and double-dose RBCs Table 9.4. However, during this study the use of polyspecific AHG was likely responsible for the detection of some 400 clinically insignificant antibodies (Steiner 1986).

Conclusions

As can be inferred from the preceding discussion, an ideal antibody detection method which would detect only, and all clinically significant antibodies, would not entail use of expensive equipment or reagents and would be simple and quick to perform. No current method fulfills either of the first two requirements. Consequently, any technique that meets the relatively general requirements of the Standards of the AABB (Holland & Schmidt 1987) is acceptable. The impact of any changes in test methods must be related to the necessary balance between increased operational costs and enhancement of patient care.

Autocontrol – direct antiglobulin test

An autocontrol, or direct antiglobulin test (DAT), is a prime example of an optional test that is widely utilized in pretransfusion studies. The test has been used to screen patients for clinically unsuspected autoimmune disease and to detect early manifestations of an immune response to previous recent transfusions.

Approximately 15% of blood samples submitted to our laboratory in 1978 for pretransfusion test had a positive DAT when polyspecific AHG was used (Judd et al 1980). In an attempt to reduce the workload associated with evaluating positive tests, we limited serological investigation to samples from patients who had been transfused within the previous three weeks, patients who were anaemic for reasons other than blood loss and patients whose serum contained concomitant unexpected antibodies. Following our 1980 report, we modified our protocol by using anti-IgG for the pretransfusion DAT and restricting serological evaluation to those patients who had been transfused within the preceding two weeks. Recently we analyzed 29-months of experience with this procedure (Judd et al 1986). Of 65 049 samples tested with anti-IgG, 3570 (5.49%) were positive but further evaluation was necessary on only 778 samples.

Reactive eluates were obtained on 260 samples and in 52 instances, were associated with alloantibodies; however, only six of these were detected in samples with nonreactive pretransfusion antibody screening tests. A further three potentially clinically significant alloantibodies, not found by elution, were detected in serum studies performed as part of the evaluation of a positive DAT.

We subjected these data to predictive value (PV) analysis (Galen & Gambino 1975). 'True-positives' were those nine samples containing potentially clinically significant alloantibodies detected solely through evaluation of a positive DAT; 'true-negatives' were 3133 of the 3570 IgG DAT-positive samples with negative screening tests for unexpected antibodies. Therefore, the PV of a positive DAT in the absence of unexpected antibodies is $9 \div 3133 \times 100 = 0.29\%$. Our experience led us to abandon the pretransfusion DAT in June 1984.

The crossmatch

In the late 1970s protocols for pretransfusion testing of surgical patients such a Type and Screen (T&S) (Boral & Henry 1977) and Maximal Surgical Blood Order Schedules (MSBOS) were advocated (Mintz et al 1976, Freidman et al 1976). T&S protocols restrict preoperative pretransfusion testing to ABO, Rh and antibody detection tests with performance of the crossmatch only when blood is actually required for transfusion. Use of a MSBOS limits the number of units crossmatched to those which predictably will be transfused for a given surgical procedure. Subsequent studies (Boral & Henry 1977, Oberman et al 1978) indicated minimal risk of missing a clinically significant antibody when a T&S was performed together with an immediate-spin (IS) crossmatch. This led to proposals for abbreviation of pretransfusion testing by omission of 37°C incubating and subsequent testing by the indirect antiglobulin test (IAT) (Garratty 1982).

The antiglobulin crossmatch became optional following actions of the Blood Products Advisory Committee of the Food and Drug Administration, and stemmed from data, including our own (Oberman et al 1978, Oberman et al 1982), similar to that shown in Table 9.3. Currently, omission of the antiglobulin crossmatch is considered appropriate for all patients except those known to have unexpected antibodies to red cell antigens (Holland & Schmidt 1987).

Analysis of the data shown in Table 9.3 yields a PV of 13% for 17 clinically significant antibodies among 131 positive crossmatches with nonreactive screening tests. Comparing this with the PV of 0.29% obtained above for the pretransfusion DAT, the greater risk is clearly associated with abbreviation of the crossmatch. Accordingly, we have recommended that institutions wishing to reduce serological testing first consider abandoning the DAT before eliminating the antiglobulin phase of the crossmatch. Indeed, we did not implement the latter procedural change until 15 months after abandoning the pretransfusion DAT.

Personnel considerations

As noted earlier, the most significant element in laboratory costs is personnel. Consolidation of effort, streamlining of required test protocols, elimination of unnecessary testing and implementation of automation are strategies for reduction of personnel.

Efficient management of personnel and appropriate staffing can be facilitated through comparison of laboratory workload statistics. Reduction or realignments of staffing should be considered when specific areas of the laboratory have a low intensity of workload. On the other hand, excessive overtime should be avoided. If an area of the laboratory consistently is subject to overtime pay, the staffing pattern of the entire laboratory should be reassessed to determine whether schedule modifications can avoid the problem.

An additional factor in conserving personnel costs is the appropriateness of employee classification, as this is invariably linked to compensation. Each position should be reviewed to determine whether the job performed corresponds to the training and pay grade of the employee. Obviously, some functions require a greater degree of skill and education than do others, and their performance should be associated with a higher job classification with correspondingly higher pay. Tasks that are repetitive and require minimum thought might well be undertaken by on-the-job trainees. For example, certain aspects of donor interviewing and testing of donor bloods can be undertaken by such individuals at lower cost than when done by technologists or nurses. At the same time it must be remembered that lack of employee versatility, and the additional supervision required, may compromise personnel savings.

SUMMARY

Clinical laboratories, including blood banks, must pay particular attention to cost-conservation, as this directly influences overall hospital costs. Streamlining laboratory testing with constant inquiry into its relevance and impact on patient care is essential. In addition, continued centralization of blood collection and processing should ensure maximal use of a limited resource and ultimately prove financially beneficial to area institutions. Alternative revenue sources also should be sought, including such blood bank-related functions as paternity testing, therapeutic plasma exchange and outpatient transfusion programmes. However, the most important factor in reducing health-care costs is reduction of personnel. This can best be achieved by their efficient use, introduction of computerization and automation, and streamlining test protocols. Nevertheless, in the enthusiasm of reducing costs, one must not lose sight of the overriding need to maintain optimal quality of patient care. Accordingly, every proposal for cost containment must always be evaluated with regard to its potential impact on patient welfare.

REFERENCES

Beck M L, Marsh W L 1977 Complement and the antiglobulin test (letter). Transfusion 17:529

Boral L I, Henry J B The type and screen: a safe alternative and supplement in selected surgical procedures 1977 Transfusion 17: 163–8

College of American Pathologists 1984 Workload recording method. Chicago

Commission of Inspection and Accreditation 1985 Inspection checklist Section V, Blood bank. College of American Pathologists, Chicago

Food and Drug Administration 1984 Code of Federal Regulations (21-CFR), part 600. Rockville Office of Biologics

Freidman B A, Oberman H A, Chadwick A R, Kindgon K I 1976 The maximum surgical blood order schedule and surgical blood use in the United States. Transfusion 16: 380–7

Galen, R S, Gambino, S R 1975 Beyond normality: the predictive value and efficacy of medical diagnoses. New York: John Wiley & Sons

Garratty G 1982 The role of compatibility tests. Transfusion 22: 169–72

Garratty G 1985 The significance of complement in immunohematology. CRC Crit. Review. Clinical Laboratory Science 20: 25–56

Holland P V, Schmidt P J 1987 Standards for blood banks and transfusion services, 12th edn. American Association of Blood Banks, Arlington, VA

Howard J E, Winn L C, Gottleib C E, Grumet F C, Garratty G, Petz L D 1982 Clinical significance of the anti-complement component of antiglobulin antisera. Transfusion 22: 269–72

Issitt P D 1979 Serology and genetics of the Rhesus blood group system. Montgomery Scientific Publications, Miami

Issitt P D 1985 Applied blood group serology, 3rd. edn Miami: Montgomery Scientific Publications

Judd W J, Butch S H, Oberman H A, Steiner E A, Bauer R C 1980 The evaluation of a positive direct antiglobulin test in pretranfusion testing. Transfusion 20: 17–23

Judd W J, Barnes B A, Steiner E A, Oberman H A, Averill D B, Butch S H 1986 The evaluation of a positive direct antiglobulin test (autocontrol) in pretransfusion testing revised. Transfusion 26: 220–224

Lalezari P, Jiang A F 1980 The manual Polybrene test: a simple and rapid test for detection of red cell antibodies. Transfusion 20: 206–11

Mintz P D, Nordine R B, Henry J B, Webb W R 1976 Expected hemotherapy in elective surgery. New York State Journal of Medicine 76: 532–7

Mollison, P L 1983 Blood transfusion in Clinical medicine, 7th Edn. Blackwell, Oxford

Moore C, Mollison P L 1976 Use of a low-ionic strength medium in manual tests for antibody detection. Transfusion 16: 291–6

Oberman H A, Barnes B A, Friedman B A 1978 The risk of abbreviating the major crossmatch in urgent or massive transfusion. Transfusion 18: 137–41

Oberman H A, Barnes B A, Steiner E A 1982 Role of the crossmatch in testing for serologic incompatibility. Transfusion 22: 12–16

Perryman M 1982 Cost accounting for test procedures. In: Karni K R, Viskochil K R, Amos P A (eds) Clinical laboratory management. Little, Brown & Co, Boston, p 345–61

Riglin H M, Patten E 1985 Enzyme-treated red cells are not cost-effective for routine pretransfusion antibody detection. Transfusion 25:453

Shulman I A, Nelson J M, Okamoto M, Malone S A 1985 Dependence of anti-Jk[a] detection on screening cell zygosity

Steiner E A 1986 Personal communication

Trudeau L R, Judd W J, Butch S H, Oberman H A 1983 Is a room-temperature crossmatch necessary for the detection of ABO errors? Transfusion 23: 237–239

Widmann F K 1985 Technical manual, 9th Edn. American Association of Blood Banks, Arlington, Va

Wright M S, Issitt P D 1979 Anticomplement and the indirect antiglobulin test test. Transfusion 19: 688–94

Transfusion support in bone marrow transplantation

INTRODUCTION

Improvements in supportive care have in part been responsible for the increased success in treating patients with cancer or other haematologic disorders. These improvements have allowed the use of very intensive chemotherapeutic and radiotherapy regimens which produce prolonged marrow suppression. Marrow transplantation, simply stated, is an extreme example of transfusion support whereby marrow (autologous or allogeneic) is used to replace marrow that has been permanently destroyed by disease or the effects of chemoradiotherapy. Marrow transplantation could not succeed, however, without readily available blood products for the temporary support of patients until the marrow graft is functioning.

Adequate transfusion support of patients undergoing marrow transplantation requires a close association between the clinical transplant service and a blood bank. A wide range of blood products and services must be available 24 hours a day and within a few minutes' notice. Additionally, the blood bank must possess certain specialized equipment such as a blood irradiator and cytapheresis devices with personnel trained to use them.

Preliminary Considerations

Patients who are candidates for marrow transplantation should be given special care when transfusions are indicated. In contrast to solid organ transplantation, studies in animals and humans have shown that transfusions from unrelated donors given prior to marrow grafting may sensitize the recipient against the marrow donor and result in graft rejection. In the clinical setting this effect is most apparent in patients with aplastic anaemia (Storb et al 1977). Patients with aplastic anaemia who have been transfused before marrow transplant have only a 50–65% survival due primarily to graft rejection and graft-versus-host-disease (GVHD). In contrast non-transfused patients with aplastic anaemia have up to an 80% survival (Storb et al 1980).

Rejection is presumed to occur because of sensitization to minor histocompatibility antigens. Indeed host lymphocytes reactive against donor cells have been found in the blood of patients with aplastic anaemia who have rejected HLA-identical grafts (Warren et al 1978). Rejection may in part be overcome by the administration of peripheral blood lymphocytes from the donor but with a concomitant increase in GVHD. It is rare for patients with haematologic malignancies to reject an HLA-identical transplant despite multiple previous transfusions. This is presumably due to the greater immunosuppression these patients receive as preparation for transplant but may also reflect immunodeficiency from their primary disease. Some have advocated the use of frozen, washed or leukocyte-poor blood products as a means of preventing graft rejection. Data from several animal studies suggest that this can be effective but there are no such studies in human marrow transplantation (Deeg et al 1981). Transfusions from family members are to be avoided in any patient who is a potential transplant recipient because of the possibility of sensitization to minor histocompatibility antigens within the family.

Marrow transplant patients may develop GVHD from viable lymphocytes contained in blood transfusions. Therefore any transfusion products which could contain viable lymphoid cells (red cells, granulocytes, platelets) must receive gamma irradiation of from 15–30 Gy in order to abolish lymphocyte proliferation (Leitman 1985). Blood product irradiation should begin with initiation of the transplant regimen and should continue for one year after transplant or longer if the patient has chronic GVHD. Commercially available caesium irradiators are available that have been specifically designed for blood product irradiation.

Because GVHD has been described in patients with haematologic malignancies or immunodeficiency diseases not receiving marrow transplants it is probably wise to give all such patients irradiated blood products (Weiden et al 1981). Obvious exceptions to this rule include not irradiating the donor marrow prior to infusion and not irradiating buffy coat transfusions given to sensitized patients with aplastic anaemia in order to reduce graft rejection. It is important to remember that any nonautologous blood transfusions given to the marrow donor before or during the marrow harvest (including buffy coat harvest) must also be irradiated to prevent the transfer of viable lymphocytes to the patient.

Although blood product support for patients undergoing marrow transplantation is similar to supportive care for patients receiving intensive chemotherapy for leukaemia, the duration of marrow aplasia is often 1–2 weeks longer. Also, the level of aplasia is usually much more profound as evidenced by peripheral blood granulocyte levels of zero. Transplant patients receiving allogeneic marrow are prone to unique complications such as GVHD that increase the need for blood transfusions. Drugs given to prevent or treat GVHD have been shown to delay engraftment of red cells or platelets, thus prolonging the need for transfusion support. In patients with chronic myelogenous leukaemia, other factors, such as the presence or absence of a spleen affect the time to engraftment and the need for transfusions (Banaji et al 1986).

RED BLOOD CELL TRANSFUSIONS AND ABO COMPATIBILITY

Red blood cell (RBC) support is most often given in the form of packed irradiated cells that have reduced levels of plasma and platelets and are prepared from unrelated random donors. Whole blood transfusions are usually given only for massive bleeding when volume replacement is needed. Frozen, washed RBC's are very expensive and rarely indicated. In most transplants the donor and recipient are ABO compatible, making RBC transfusion support fairly straightforward.

It seems reasonable to give RBC transfusions frequently enough to maintain a haematocrit of about 30%. One may calculate that a normal 70 kg adult, producing no RBCs should require approximately one unit of RBC per week or about 7 units per transplant to maintain a 25–30% haematocrit. Data from Seattle indicate that patients require on average 10–18 units per transplant and that patients with relapsed leukaemia or CML need more units compared to patients with aplastic anaemia or leukaemia in remission (Storb 1981). Additionally we have found that patients receiving cyclosporine A for GVHD prophylaxis had a significantly increased RBC transfusion requirement compared with patients receiving methotrexate (Deeg et al 1985).

In about 15–20% of HLA-identical donor recipient pairs major ABO incompatibility exists (Bensinger et al 1982). In this situation the recipient's plasma contains anti-A or anti-B antibodies directed against donor RBC. In minor ABO incompatibility the donor plasma contains anti-RBC antibodies against recipient cells. It has been shown that the ABO system is not an important marrow transplantation antigen either for graft rejection or GVHD. Host antibody does not influence engraftment because primitive haematopoetic stem cells do not express ABO blood group antigens. Similarly donor antibody does not lead to GVHD because host non-RBC tissues do not make ABO antigens. However when the marrow transplant recipient's plasma contains a sufficient quantity of antibodies directed against ABO group antigens of the donor red cells, there is the risk of a haemolytic transfusion reaction at the time of marrow infusion. We have determined that when the recipient's anti-RBC titre is 1 : 16 or less, it is safe to infuse whole, unmodified marrow.

To avoid haemolysis, a number of techniques have been used including modification of donor marrow to deplete red cells, removal of recipient antibodies by apheresis procedures or a combination of the two. Red cell depletion may be accomplished by bag centrifugation (Falkenburg et al 1985), gravity sedimentation (Dinsmore et al 1983), and semi-automated equipment such as red cell washers (Blacklock et al 1982), continuous-flow

(Sniecinski et al 1985) or intermittent flow (Braine et al 1982) blood cell separators. Most of the above techniques are rendered more efficient by the addition of red cell sedimenting agents such as dextran or hydroxyethyl starch.

All depletion techniques are effective at removing red cells and avoiding haemolysis but result in some loss of mononuclear cells. This is usually not a problem when patients have an HLA-identical sibling and undergo the heavy immunosuppression required for treatment of malignant disease. However, transplants performed for aplastic anaemia or from HLA mismatched donors have higher rejection rates. In these situations the loss of stem cells during RBC depletion may jeopardize engraftment. The use of ficoll-metrizoate in combination with a semi-automated cell washer is not recommended because of higher than normal mononuclear cell losses with possible subsequent failure to engraft in some patients (Hill personal communication).

Removal of recipient antibodies can be effectively performed with plasma exchange or immunoadsorptive techniques (Bensinger 1984). Plasma exchange uses continuous-flow or intermittent-flow blood cell separators or plasma membrane filtration devices. Replacement fluids consist of 5% albumin solution and fresh-frozen, cyroprecipitate-poor plasma. Plasma exchange is effective but drawbacks include expense, allergic reactions and exposure to infectious agents from plasma. We have utilized immuno-adsorption by linking synthetically manufactured blood group antigens to a solid support. Recipient plasma or whole blood can be perfused through the columns continuously in order to remove the antibody. Immuno-adsorption is slightly less efficient compared to plasma exchange for removing antibodies but the difference is not clinically significant. All apheresis procedures do result in some loss of platelets due to removal or activation.

In major ABO incompatibility, blood components given prior to trans-plant should be of recipient type. Packed RBC's generally do not contain enough plasma to be of consequence but platelet concentrates should have excess plasma removed in order to avoid the passive transfusion of anti-RBC antibodies. During the post-transplant phase recipient or group O RBCs should be given until recipient antibody to donor cells is no longer detect-able. This averages 30 days with a range of 2–120 days. Persistence of anti-RBC antibody of donor type has been associated with delayed production of RBCs and prolonged transfusion requirements. Donor type platelets should be given post-transplant.

In minor ABO incompatibility, recipient type RBCs and platelets should be given prior to transplant. Removal of plasma from the marrow of donors with antibodies against the recipient's RBC type is necessary only for titres greater than 1 : 64, when dilution of donor plasma after infusion would be insufficient to avoid haemolysis. After transplant donor type RBC's and recipient type platelets or reduced volume donor type platelets should be given until recipient type red cells are no longer detectable in the circulation. As in major ABO incompatibility, studies indicate that minor ABO incompatibility is not associated with an increased risk of graft rejection or GVHD.

The simultaneous occurrence of major and minor ABO is a rare event. If an apheresis procedure is used for removing donor directed isohaemagglutinins, it will be necessary to remove plasma from the donor marrow should the anti-recipient isohaemagglutinins be high enough. If red cell depletion is used, sufficient donor plasma will also be removed to avoid haemolysis. For RBC support, group O cells should be used. Platelets should be blood group AB or have excess plasma removed. Plasma, if needed, should be blood group AB.

PLASMA AND PLASMA DERIVED PRODUCT TRANSFUSIONS

The chemoradiotherapy regimens used in transplantation cause severe nausea, vomiting, diarrhoea and mucositis. After transplantation, infection, GVHD and organ toxicity with resulting dysfunction contribute to persistence of these symptoms. Hypoalbuminaemia is a frequent finding and this along with increased vascular permeability may aggravate such conditions as veno-occlusive disease of the liver and pulmonary fluid overload. Thus, marrow transplant patients frequently require albumin or plasma transfusions after transplant because of their severe catabolic condition. Plasma transfusions should be compatible with both donor and recipient cells. Incompatible plasma infusions have been reported to produce a fatal respiratory distress syndrome associated with the pulmonary deposition of agglutinated red cells. Similar problems have been described after transfusion of plasma containing anti-leukocyte antibodies.

Since it has been known that patients may have impaired regulation of immunoglobulin synthesis after transplant, there has been an increased interest in the transfusion of immunoglobulin preparations during the transplant period as a means of decreasing the incidence of bacterial and viral infections. High titre cytomegalovirus (CMV) immunoglobulin or plasma has been shown in some studies to decrease CMV infections after transplant (Winston et al 1984). CMV immunoglobulin used at this centre was less effective at preventing CMV infection than CMV seronegative blood products (Bowden et al 1986) but did decrease the incidence of post transplant septicemia in the first 100 days (Petersen, personal communication).

PLATELET TRANSFUSIONS

The use of platelet transfusions has significantly decreased the morbidity and mortality associated with thrombocytopaenia. The most widely used type of platelets for transfusion are obtained by centrifugal separation from units of whole blood donated by random volunteers. Most blood banks separate whole blood into component parts consisting of packed RBCs, plasma, platelets and in some cases, cryoprecipitate. The platelet rich plasma obtained from one unit is further centrifuged in order to obtain a 50–100 ml volume containing the platelets. Platelets are stored as single units, at room temperature and with constant agitation until needed. Newer plastic bags that permit better gas exchange and pH stability have extended the ability to store platelets from three to five or seven days (Murphy et al 1982). When needed platelets from 4–8 separate units are pooled and transfused within eight hours of donation.

While studies have shown that ABO incompatible platelets produce about a 20% lower increment compared to ABO compatible platelets the difference is not clinically significant (Duquesnoy et al 1979). The major risk of such transfusions is the passive acquistion of antibodies against donor or recipient RBC's leading to haemolysis. Therefore it is desirable to reduce the quantity of plasma in the incompatible pooled platelets by an extra centrifugation step.

An important advance in platelet transfusion therapy has been the development of blood cell separator equipment which permits the collection of four or more units of platelets from single donors. With these machines family members or HLA-selected, unrelated donors can be used for platelet support when patients become alloimmunized to platelets pooled from random donors. Several types of equipment are available that vary in complexity and automation. One can choose simpler intermittent-flow devices that only require a single venepuncture for collection. Although these machines are the least expensive to purchase they require more operator attention while running and the collection time is longer. Continuous flow devices collect the same number of platelets in less time but require two venepunctures and are expensive to purchase.

The obvious reason for transfusing platelets is to control overt bleeding in a thrombocytopaenic patient with active haemorrhage. When to give platelets for the prophylaxis of bleeding is less clear. While there is a direct relationship between the bleeding time and platelet count for levels below $100\,000/\mu l$ clinically significant bleeding does not occur until much lower levels. Previous studies measuring ^{51}Cr stool blood loss in thrombocytopaenic patients have indicated that at a platelet count of 5–$10\,000/\mu l$ spontaneous bleeding occurs (Slichter et al 1978). However certain drug therapies such as antibiotics and prednisone were found to have a marked effect on enhancing gastrointestinal blood loss. Most clinical studies of prophylactic platelet transfusions have indicated that 15–$20\,000/\mu l$ is a more appropriate level to transfuse although it is acknowledged that individual patients vary greatly in their tendency to bleed at any given platelet level.

In stable patients that have no underlying structural problems that would increase the likelihood of bleeding we monitor platelet counts once a day and transfuse platelets for counts of less than $20\,000/\mu l$. Adult patients receive 6–8 units of platelets pooled from random donors with each transfusion. Paediatric patients are given 4 units if less than 30 kg. For patients of less than 15 kg, it is usually necessary to remove excess plasma from the platelets to avoid volume overload. Patients who become refractory to random donor platelets may require support from family members or HLA-matched unrelated donors (see Alloimmunization).

The success of a platelet transfusion may be judged by the increase in the platelet count obtained one and 24 hours after transfusion. The corrected count increment (CCI) uses the body surface area of the patient normalized for the number of platelets transfused according to the following formula (Klein 1982):

$$CCI = \frac{(\text{Post-transfusion count} - \text{Pre-transfusion count})}{\text{Number of platelets transfused} \times 10^{11}} \times \text{Body surface area (M}^2)$$

An average unit containing 0.7×10^{11} platelets should produce an absolute increment of $10\,000/\mu l$ in a 70 kg adult (blood volume = 6 litres) and a CCI = 18 000 (surface area = 1.8 m^2) if recovery were 100%. Actual studies using fresh, radiochromium labelled platelets have demonstrated a recovery of 65% due to splenic sequestration of about 1/3 of platelets (Peters, et al 1980). The CCI has clearly been shown to correlate with control of bleeding although studies are not available on its relationship to platelets used for bleeding prophylaxis. Patients who achieve one hour post transfusion CCIs of less than 10% predicted to two consecutive transfusions are considered to be platelet refractory.

In an analysis of platelet support for patients undergoing HLA-matched transplantation for acute nonlymphocytic leukaemia (ANL) or chronic myelogenous leukaemia (CML) platelet refractory patients required significantly more units of platelets after transplantation, primarily from family members and HLA-matched community donors. As might be expected, patients who took longer to engraft required more days and more units of platelet support than patients who engrafted earlier. Factors that did not influence speed of engraftment included marrow cell dose, patient age or sex, pre-transplant conditioning or refractoriness to random donor platelets. The most important risk factor for delayed engraftment was the drug used for GVHD prophylaxis and the development of GVHD. Methotrexate given to patients post-transplant to prevent GVHD had a significant delay on time to engraft platelets and granulocytes compared to patients treated with cyclosporine (Deeg et al 1985).

43 of 186 patients transplanted for ANL became platelet transfusion dependent for a second time after at least a week of no longer requiring platelet transfusions. 88% of those patients developed grade 2 or greater GVHD. While refractoriness to random donor platelets makes support of thrombocytopaenic patients more difficult, it does not prolong the time of support.

GRANULOCYTE TRANSFUSIONS

The preparative regimens used in marrow transplantation result in periods of profound granulocytopaenia ranging from 2–4 weeks. Many studies in patients undergoing chemotherapy for leukaemia indicate an increased risk of infection at granulocyte levels below $1000/\mu$l with more serious infections such as sepsis becoming a problem below $500/\mu$l. With the success of platelet transfusions in preventing haemorrhage of thrombocytopaenic patients and the availability of techniques for collecting large numbers of granulocytes for transfusion it seemed reasonable to attempt similar interventions to treat and prevent infection.

Normal daily production of granulocytes has been estimated at 10^{11} for an average sized adult. Actual blood pool levels are one-half this amount (5×10^{10}). Another 4×10^{11} granulocytes are available for release from the bone marrow reserves. Initial clinical reports of transfusion therapy utilized granulocytes collected from patients with CML which yielded as many as 1.8×10^{11} granulocytes (Freireich et al 1964). Transfusion of these cells often gave dramatic clinical results and it was possible to demonstrate that transfused cells migrated to sites of infection. With the development of semi-automated blood cell processors the popularity of granulocyte transfusions increased but even with RBC sedimentating agents, arteriovenous shunts and corticosteroids it is only possible to collect 1–1.5×10^{10} granulocytes from normal donors. This is about 2% of the neutrophils available to an individual with normal marrow function and less than one-tenth the quantity collected from donors with CML. This disparity in dosage of cells may explain in part why the promising results attained initially were never fully realized. In general most studies have suffered from small numbers of patients, using relatively modest numbers of granulocytes (less than 10^{10}) and perhaps most importantly, using unrelated, unmatched donors leading to relatively rapid alloimmunization.

Devices available for granulocyte collection include several models of continuous-flow cell centrifuges which have the highest collection efficiency, and intermittent-flow devices which are less costly and simpler to use. Gravity sedimentation is too cumbersome and inefficient to be used routinely. Concerns about donor safety, patient transfusion reactions and product efficacy have made filtration leukapheresis techniques obsolete.

One of the earliest studies using normal donors compared the addition of granulocyte transfusions to appropriate antibiotics alone for established septicemia in patients with granulocyte counts below $500/\mu$l due to a variety of causes. Although there was no significant difference in survival between the two groups, a subgroup of patients who survived long enough to receive at least 4 transfusions had a better ultimate survival than a similar subgroup among controls (Graw et al 1972). This study is also important because it was one of the first to indicate that HLA matching and anti-leukocyte antibodies have an important influence on granulocyte recovery.

Three later studies evaluated prospectively granulocytes added to an antibiotic regimen in patients with neutropenia related to treatment for leukaemia and either fever, documented sepsis or fever and sepsis unresponsive to an antibiotic trial (Alavi et al 1977, Herzig et al 1977, Vogler 1977). All indicated that granulocytes were more effective at treating documented infection and that, as one might expect, marrow recovery had the greatest impact on survival. Two randomized prospective studies have evaluated prophylactic granulocytes in marrow transplant patients with granulocyte levels below 500 or $200/\mu l$ and without the use of prophylactic systemic antibiotics (Clift et al 1978, Winston et al 1980). Both studies indicated less septicemia in the transfused group although one was not significant. While one of the studies used family members or the marrow donor for support the other used unrelated donors for transfusions which may have compromised the results.

Most of the arguments to use or not use granulocyte transfusions for infection prophylaxis have become moot in view of improvements in antibiotic therapy and recognition of the hazards of granulocyte transfusions. A recent study comparing prophylactic systemic antibiotics to prophylactic granulocytes found no difference in infection rates (Petersen F, personal communication). Alloimmunization is a frequent complication of granulocyte transfusions, and can lead to fevers, pulmonary infiltrates and an acute respiratory distress syndrome (Schiffer et al 1979, Wright et al 1981). Furthermore investigators have come to recognize that granulocyte transfusions from CMV positive donors increase the risks of CMV infection (Hersman et al 1982).

Such observations and cost effectiveness issues have caused us to change our patterns of granulocyte use over the past eight years (Rosenshein et al 1980). We no longer use granulocyte transfusions prophylactically in marrow transplant patients. Instead we reserve granulocyte support for patients with documented, persistent serious infections such as sepsis or parenchymal lesions, granulocyte counts below $200/\mu l$, and failure to respond to at least 3 days of appropriate antibiotic therapy. One additional group of patients who may benefit from daily granulocyte transfusions are those patients with established infection at the time of transplantation.

Donors are selected from family members in order to minimize the development of alloimmunity. We perform daily granulocyte collections with the selected donor utilizing a continuous flow cell centrifuge. Blood access is obtained with a double lumen Hickman central venous catheter. We use hydroxyethyl starch as a sedimenting agent but do not use steroids because of the risk of daily administration to a single donor. Transfusions continue until the patient's endogenous granulocyte level begins to rise above a level of $250–500/\mu l$.

ALLOIMMUNIZATION

An important consequence of repeated blood product transfusions is the development of alloimmunization. Alloimmunity may develop to red cell antigens but is more often directed against leukocyte and platelet associated histocompatibility antigens. Clinically this is characterized by graft rejection or the failure to achieve useful increments to transfusions of platelets pooled from random donors or to achieve useful granulocyte increments after granulocyte transfusions (refractoriness).

In patients with leukaemia undergoing induction chemotherapy, up to 50% become refractory to platelets from random donors by four or fewer transfusions (Dutcher et al 1981). Lymphocytotoxicity testing suggests that most of these patients are alloimmunized. Data from our centre suggest that the problem of platelet refractoriness is at least as great in marrow transplant recipients.

We have examined the incidence of refractoriness to platelets pooled from random donors in patients with ANL in first remission and CML in chronic phase undergoing allogeneic marrow transplantation. In 186 patients with ANL 6% were refractory to their first transfusions from random donors and an additional 39% became refractory during the post-transplant phase. Of 67 individuals with CML, 11% were refractory to random donor platelets initially and an additional 35% became refractory after transplant. Splenectomized patients with CML became platelet refractory far less frequently (6%) than patients transplanted with intact spleens (67%), making platelet support easier (Banaji et al 1986).

Data from our own blood centre indicate that platelet refractory patients require significantly more resources than nonrefractory patients. In a one month period 273 patients required 5900 units of platelets. Of these, 22 patients required at least 5 consecutive daily platelet transfusions, mostly for alloimmunization. These 22 patients represented only 8% of the transfused population yet utilized 35% (2042) of the platelets.

In defining the problem of alloimmunization it is important to identify other causes of platelet refractoriness. Multiple problems causing increased platelet consumption that exist in patients undergoing marrow transplantation include fever, sepsis, splenomegaly, drug therapy, disseminated intravascular coagulation, malignancy and active haemorrhage. The CCI measured one hour after transfusion is the most useful indicator of alloimmunization (Daly et al 1980). However recent studies suggest that consumptive factors can prevent useful platelet increments (McFarland et al 1982). Thus the CCI must be interpreted with caution in the presence of clinical conditions that may cause increased consumption.

Platelet associated antibody tests can help support a diagnosis of alloimmunization but no single test is sufficiently sensitive or specific. Some investigators have relied on lymphocytotoxic antibodies, but this is controversial (Hogge et al 1983). A reduction in fibrinogen survival is often observed in patients with platelet consumption. However, we have noted that patients with leukaemia in remission who have normal platelet counts may have a reduced fibrinogen survival presumably from their existing disease.

In patients who are platelet refractory due to alloimmunization we frequently utilize family members or the marrow donor during the post transplant phase. Pre-transplant, or if family donors are not available during the post-transplant period, it may be necessary to rely on HLA-matched community donors for support. Studies have indicated that the degree of HLA matching closely correlates with success of the transfusion. However some studies have indicated that even fully HLA matched platelets from unrelated donors fail to circulate in up to 35% of alloimmunized patients (Slichter 1980). Studies performed at this centre indicate that with a pool of 500 community donors useful donors were located for 31 of 34 patients refractory to random donor platelets. Only 68% of fully matched platelets gave successful transfusion responses, in part due to consumptive factors. Platelet crossmatch tests gave a 63% predictability of the transfusion response (McFarland 1982).

Two relatively new approaches have been reported for refractory or alloimmunized patients. High dose intravenous immunoglobulin has been reported to be useful for reversing alloimmunization in several studies, although a randomized study showed no benefit (Schiffer et al 1984). We have plasma exchanged 18 patients who were platelet refractory and observed improved post-transfusion increments in eleven patients (Bensinger et al 1986). However this was not a randomized study and patients were not all clearly alloimmunized.

Since methods for dealing with alloimmunization are not uniformly successful, efforts have focused on trying to prevent alloimmunization from occurring. Prospective studies of patients undergoing induction therapy for acute leukaemia have suggested that therapeutic platelet transfusions when compared to prophylactic transfusions halved the number of units of plate-lets required with similar numbers of bleeding days and deaths in each group. However it is not clear that limiting the number of units of platelets transfused will prevent patients from becoming alloimmunized. Dutcher et al found no relationship between the number of units of platelets transfused and the percentage of patients who became alloimmunized (Dutcher et al 1981). Alternatively alloimmunization could be prevented by limiting antigen exposure as in the use of single donors or by modification of the transfusion product.

Two studies have compared the use of platelets from single unrelated donors, either partially HLA-matched or random, with platelets pooled from random donors for support of patients with leukaemia undergoing induction therapy or marrow transplantation. Although both studies suggested that single donor transfusions decreased the rate of alloimmuniz-ation and platelet refractoriness, one study used leukocyte depleted RBCs in both groups which may have had an important influence (see Table 10.1). In any case no study has really compared platelets from single unrelated donors to platelets pooled from random donors in a prospective, randomized fashion for patients undergoing marrow transplantation.

Table 10.1 Prevention of alloimmunization with leukocyte depleted blood products.

	Experimental				Control			
Investigator	Platelets WBC/U $\times 10^6$	Type +	LP RBC*	% ALLO #	Platelets WBC/U $\times 10^6$	Type +	LP RBC*	% ALLO #
Eernisee[1]	1	R	Y	25	450	R	N	95
Slichter[2]	3	R	Y	25	50	R	N	50
Schiffer[3]	12	R	Y	20	65	R	N	42
Gmur[4]	60	SD	Y	15	14	R	Y	40
Murphy[5]	10	SD	Y	11	100	SD	N	50

+ Type of platelets given, R = pooled random donor, SD = single donor
* Leukocyte depleted red cells given yes/no
# Percentage of recipients alloimmunized
[1] Eernisse 1981
[2] Slichter personal communication
[3] Schiffer et al 1983
[4] Gmur et al 1983
[5] Murphy et al 1986

Sensitization is believed to result from leukocyte contamination in red cells and platelet concentrates that are transfused. Indeed studies have shown that leukocyte transfusions from unrelated donors are highly immunogenic. Data from animal studies suggest that blood transfusions given to mice or dogs prior to histocompatible marrow grafting result in a very high rate of graft rejection. If however, red cells or platelets depleted of leukocytes are given, no graft rejection is observed (Storb et al 1979, Deeg et al 1981).

These data are of interest because while RBCs lack all histocompatibility antigens, platelets are known to carry class I but not class II antigens. It has been postulated that class II antigen carrying cells are a necessary component in transfusions for the recognition of class I antigens. Such cells may provide 'antigen-presenting' function in transfused cells that leads to sensitization. Further studies in an alloimmunized dog model have suggested that by removing Ia antigen positive cells from whole blood, transfusion-induced sensitization and subsequent graft rejection could be prevented. Pure platelet preparations given to rats are non-immunogenic. Inactivation of Ia positive cells by ultraviolet light in platelet concentrates given to dogs prevented alloimmunization and platelet refractoriness (Slichter et al 1984).

While no data are available on the prevention of alloimmunization with leukocyte depleted blood products in marrow transplant recipients, there are several studies using such products in patients with leukaemia undergoing chemotherapy (Table 10.1). These studies suggest that leukocyte depleted RBC are a very important part of any prevention programme and that the addition of leukocyte depleted platelets and perhaps single donors as well may have additive beneficial effects. Such transfusion programmes are being explored in patients undergoing marrow transplantation.

INFECTIOUS COMPLICATIONS

An important hazard of intensive transfusion support is the transmission of infectious disease. The use of all volunteer blood and screening programs has all but eliminated hepatitis B. However, non-A, non-B hepatitis continues to be prevalent. The majority of patients are asymptomatic, and only liver function abnormalities are observed. This makes the diagnosis of non-A, non-B hepatitis particularly difficult in marrow transplant patients who frequently have other causes of liver dysfunction such as veno-occlusive disease, GVHD or CMV infection. The differential diagnosis of abnormal liver function tests in marrow transplant recipients often requires a liver biopsy.

CMV is the single most important opportunistic pathogen as a cause of post-marrow transplant morbidity and mortality. The virus is one of a group of herpes viruses that commonly infect man. Prevalence of infection, as measured by seropositivity, approach 100% in underdeveloped countries and range from 25–50% in industrialized nations. Once infected the virus remains in a latent form in some vital organs, most importantly bone marrow and leukocytes. Studies have shown that CMV infection after marrow transplantation is due to reactivation of endogenous virus in 30–50% of cases or primary infection from transfused blood products and bone marrow. In marrow transplant recipients CMV causes fatal interstitial pneumonia, enterocolitis, hepatitis, and oesophagitis. CMV infections also may cause significant marrow suppression after transplant leading to increased transfusion requirements (Verdonck et al 1985).

Effective treatment for interstitial pneumonitis due to CMV is presently not available. Passive immunoprophylaxis of primary CMV infection with CMV immunoglobulin has been reported to be successful for certain subgroups of marrow transplant recipients. A prophylactic study of CMV immunoglobulin conducted at UCLA showed a reduced incidence of symptomatic infections and CMV pneumonia (Winston et al 1984). Another study showed protection with CMV immunoglobulin only for patients not given granulocyte transfusions. A prospective trial in our centre of CMV immunoglobulin failed to prevent primary CMV infections in patients transplanted from CMV seropositive donors. Those patients also received blood products not screened for CMV (donor seropositivity is approximately 50%) and perhaps the immunoglobulin failed to protect because of the large amount of CMV positive blood products received. Thus the efficacy of CMV immunoglobulin probably depends on the titre of antibody and the virus load in the blood products transfused. Recent studies have demonstrated that transfusion of CMV seronegative blood products exclusively (including the transplanted bone marrow) can prevent the acquisition of primary CMV infection (Bowden et al 1986).

Granulocyte transfusions from CMV positive donors into CMV negative marrow transplant recipients have been shown to carry a high risk of disease acquisition. It is possible to culture CMV from the white cell fraction of whole blood taken from infected and even asymptomatic persons. Since it is known that leukocytes harbor CMV it has been suggested that leukocyte depleted blood products may protect against CMV infection. One study showed that the use of filtered RBC, which removes 95% of leukocytes, and centrifuged leukocyte poor platelets, with 99% removal, prevented CMV infection in 11 of 13 patients undergoing autologous marrow transplant (Verdonck et al 1985). Larger studies to test the efficacy of leukocyte depleted blood products on the prevention of CMV are underway.

SUMMARY

Adequate transfusion support is an important component to marrow transplant programmes. This requires not only expertise in blood banking but a first-hand knowledge of the clinical aspects of marrow transplantation and the need for certain specialized equipment such as a blood irradiator. RBC and platelet support requires information on donor and recipient ABO types and anti-RBC titres. Transfusion programmes using only platelets pooled from random donors are probably insufficient due to frequent platelet refractoriness and alloimmunization. Platelets are often required from family members and community donors. Prophylactic granulocyte transfusions have probably been made obsolete by the recognition of their hazards and improvements in antibiotic therapy. However, there is still a role for granulocyte support in selected patients with resistant infections and a suitable donor. Newer transfusion programmes are underway that will address the most important hazards of blood products, alloimmunization and CMV transmission.

REFERENCES

Alavi J B, Root R K, Djerassi I, Evans A E et al 1977 A randomized clinical trial of granulocyte transfusions for infection in acute leukemia. New England Journal of Medicine 296: 706–711
Banaji M, Bearman S I, Buckner C D et al 1986 The effects of splenectomy on engraftment and platelet transfusion requirements in patients with chronic myelogenous leukemia undergoing marrow transplantation. American Journal of Hematology 22: 275–283
Bensinger W I 1984 Selective removal of A and B isoagglutinins. In: Pineda A A ed. Selective Plasma Component Removal. Futura Publishing, Mount Kisco, NY pp 43–70
Bensinger W I, Buckner C D, Clift R A, Slichter S J, Thomas E D 1986 Plasma exchange for platelet alloimmunization. Transplantation 41: 602–605
Bensinger W I, Buckner C D, Thomas E D, Clift R A 1982 ABO-incompatible marrow transplants. Transplantation 33: 427–429
Blacklock H A, Gilmore M J M L, Prentice H G, et al 1982 ABO-incompatible bone-marrow transplantation: Removal of red blood cells from donor marrow avoiding recipient antibody depletion. Lancet 2: 1061–1064
Bowden R A, Sayers M, Flournoy N, et al 1986 Cytomegalovirus immune globulin and seronegative blood products to prevent primary cytomegalovirus infection after marrow transplant. New England Journal of Medicine 314: 1006–1010
Braine H G, Sensenbrenner L L, Wright S K, Tutschka P J, Saral R, Santos G W 1982 Bone marrow transplantation with major ABO blood group incompatibility using erythrocyte depletion of marrow prior to infusion. Blood 60: 420–425

Clift R A, Sanders J E, Thomas E D, Williams B, Buckner C D 1978 Granulocyte transfusions for the prevention of infection in patients receiving bone-marrow transplants. New England Journal of Medicine 298: 1052–1057

Daly P A, Schiffer C A, Aisner J, Wiernik P H 1980 Platelet transfusion therapy. One-hour posttransfusion increments are valuable in predicting the need for HLA-matched preparations. Journal of American Medical Association 243: 435–438

Deeg H J, Storb R, Thomas E D et al 1985 Cyclosporine as prophylaxis for graft-versus-host disease: A randomized study in patients undergoing marrow transplantation for acute nonlymphoblastic leukemia. Blood 65: 1325–1334

Deeg H J, Torok-Storb B, Storb R, et al 1981 Rejection of DLA-identical canine littermate marrow after transfusion-induced sensitization: Antigens involved are expressed on cotton-wool adherent but not on nonadherent mononuclear cells, granulocytes or thoracic duct lymphocytes. In: Baum S J, Ledney G D, Khan A ed. Experimental Hematology Today. S. Karger, Basel pp 31–37

Dinsmore R E, Reich L M, Kapoor N et al 1983 ABH incompatible bone marrow transplantation: removal of erythrocytes by starch sedimentation. British Journal of Haematology 54: 441–449

Duquesnoy R J, Anderson A J, Tomasulo P A, Aster R H 1979 ABO compatibility and platelet transfusions of alloimmunized thrombocytopenic patients. Blood 54: 595–599

Dutcher J P, Schiffer C A, Aisner J, Wiernik P H 1981 Alloimmunization following platelet transfusion: The absence of a dose-response relationship. Blood 57: 395–398

Eernisse J G, Brand A 1981 Prevention of platelet refractoriness due to HLA antibodies by administration of leukocyte-poor blood components. Experimental Hematology 9: 77–83

Falkenburg J H F, Schaafsma M R, Jansen J et al 1985 Recovery of hematopoiesis after blood-group-incompatible bone marrow transplantation with red-blood-cell-depleted grafts. Transplantation 39: 514–520

Freireich E J, Levin R H, Whang J, Carbone P P, Bronson W, Morse E E 1964 The function and fate of transfused leukocytes from donors with chronic myelocytic leukemia in leukopenic recipients. Annals of the New York Academy of Science 113: 1081–1089

Gmur J, von Felten A, Osterwalder B et al 1983 Delayed alloimmunization using random single donor platelet transfusions: A prospective study in thrombocytopenic patients with acute leukemia. Blood 62: 473–479

Graw R G, Jr, Herzig G, Perry S, Henderson E S 1972 Normal granulocyte transfusion therapy. Treatment of septicemia due to gram-negative bacteria. New England Journal of Medicine 287: 367–371

Hersman J, Meyers J D, Thomas E D, Buckner C D, Clift R 1982 The effect of granulocyte transfusions upon the incidence of cytomegalovirus infection after allogeneic marrow transplantation. Annals of Internal Medicine 96; 149–152

Herzig R H, Herzig G P, Graw R G Jr, Bull M I, Ray K K 1977 Successful granulocyte transfusion therapy for gram-negative septicemia. A prospectively randomized controlled study. New England Journal of Medicine 296: 701–705

Hogge D E, Dutcher J P, Aisner J, Schiffer C A 1982 Lymphocytotoxic antibody is a predictor of response to random donor platelet transfusion. American Journal of Hematology 14: 363–369

Klein C A, Blajchman M A 1982 Alloantibodies and platelet destruction. Seminars in Thrombosis and Haemostasis 8: 105–115

Leitman S F, Holland P V 1985 Irradiation of blood products. Indications and guidelines. Transfusion 25: 293–300

McFarland J G, Slichter S J 1982 Support of alloimmunized patients with HLA-matched platelets. Blood 60: (Suppl 1) 180a

McFarland J G, Slichter S J, Appelbaum F 1982 Alloimmune vs. consumptive platelet 'refractorines' in AML. Blood 60 (Suppl 1): 180a

Murphy M F, Metcalfe P, Thomas H et al 1986 Use of leucocyte-poor blood components and HLA-matched-platelet donors to prevent HLA alloimmunization. British Journal of Haematology 62: 529–534

Murphy S, Kahn R A, Holme S et al 1982 Improved storage of platelets for transfusion in a new container. Blood 60: 194–200

Peters A M, Klonizakis I, Lavender J P, Lewis S M 1980 Use of [111]Indium-labelled platelets to measure spleen function. British Journal of Haematology 46: 587–593

Rosenshein M S, Farewell V T, Price T H, Larson E B, Dale D C 1980 The cost effectiveness of therapeutic and prophylactic leukocyte transfusion. New England Journal of Medicine 302: 1058–1062

Schiffer C A, Aisner J, Daly P A, Schimpff S C, Wiernik P H 1979 Alloimmunization following prophylactic granulocyte transfusion. Blood 54: 766–774

Schiffer C A, Dutcher J P, Aisner J, Hogge D, Wiernik P H, Reilly J P 1983 A randomized trial of leukocyte-depleted platelet transfusion to modify alloimmunization in patients with leukemia. Blood 62: 815–820

Schiffer C A, Hogge D E, Aisner J, Dutcher J P, Lee E J, Papenberg D 1984 High-dose intravenous gammaglobulin in alloimmunized platelet transfusion recipients. Blood 64: 937–940

Slichter S J 1980 Controversies in platelet transfusion therapy. Annual Reviews of Medicine 31: 509–540

Slichter S J, Deeg H J, Kennedy M 1984 Prevention of platelet (PLT) alloimmunization: use of cyclosporine-loaded (C–L) or UV-irradiated donor platelets. Blood 64 (Suppl. 1): 231a

Slichter S J, Harker L A 1978 Thrombocytopenia: Mechanisms and management of defects in platelet production. Clinical Haematology 7: 523–539

Sniecinski I, Henry S, Ritchey B, Branch D R, Blume K G 1985 Erythrocyte depletion of ABO-incompatible bone marrow. Journal of Clinical Apheresis 2: 231–234

Storb R, Prentice R L, Thomas E D 1977 Treatment of aplastic anemia by marrow transplantation from HLA identical siblings. Prognostic factors associated with graft versus host disease and survival. Journal of Clinical Investigation 59: 625–632

Storb R, Thomas E D, Buckner C D et al 1980 Marrow transplantation in thirty 'untransfused' patients with severe aplastic anemia. Annals of Inter Medicine 92: 30–36

Storb R, Weiden P L 1981 Transfusion problems associated with transplantion. Seminars in Haematology 18: 163–176

Storb R, Weiden P L, Deeg H J et al 1979 Rejection of marrow from DLA-identical canine littermates given transfusions before grafting: Antigens involved are expressed on leukocytes and skin epithelial cells but not on platelets and red blood cells. Blood 54: 477–484

Verdonck L F, Middeldorp J M, Kreeft H A J G, Hauw The T, Hekker A, De Gast G C 1985 Primary cytomegalovirus infection and its prevention after autologous bone marrow transplantation. Transplantation 39: 455–457

Verdonck L F, van Heugten H, De Gast 1985 Delay in platelet recovery after bone marrow transplantation: Impact of cytomegalovirus infection. Blood 66: 921–925

Vogler W R, Winton E F 1977 A controlled study of the efficacy of granulocyte transfusions in patients with neutropenia. American Journal of Medicine 63: 548–554

Warren R P, Storb R, Weiden P L, Su P J, Thomas E D 1978 Association of lymphocyte-mediated cytotoxicity (LMC) and antibody-dependent cell-mediated cytotoxicity (ADCC) with bone-marrow graft rejection in HLA- identical siblings. Transplantation Proceedings 10: 433–434

Weiden P L, Zuckerman N, Hansen J A et al 1981 Fatal graft-versus-host disease in a patient with lymphoblastic leukemia following normal granulocyte tranfusions. Blood 57: 328–332

Winston D J, Ho W G, Lin C H, Budinger M D, Champlin R E, Gale R P 1984 Intravenous immunoglobulin for modification of cytomegalovirus infections associated with bone marrow transplantation. Preliminary results of a controlled trial. American Journal of Medicine 76(3A): 128–133

Winston D J, Ho W G, Young L S, Gale R P 1980 Prophylactic granulocyte transfusions during human bone marrow transplantation. American Journal of Medicine 68: 893–897

Wright D G, Robichaud K J, Pizzo P A, Deisseroth A B 1981 Lethal pulmonary reactions associated with the combined use of amphotericin B and leukocyte transfusions. New England Journal of Medicine 304: 1185–1189

11 *D. H. Crawford   T. Azim   G. L. Daniels   E. R. Huehns*

Monoclonal antibodies to the Rh D antigen

INTRODUCTION

The requirement for anti-Rh D immunoglobulin for use in prevention of Rh haemolytic disease of the newborn and for grouping reagents is increasing, while the success of Rh immune prophylaxis programmes has led to a reduction in the natural supply of anti-Rh D. Attempts are now being made to produce suitable, monoclonal anti-Rh D in vitro. If successful this could provide an ample supply of antibody for all needs.

Historical perspectives

When in 1939, Levine and Stetson described a case of unexpected blood group incompatibility they were in fact reporting the first example of incompatibility to anti-Rh D antibody, clinically the most important blood group antibody after anti-A and anti-B (Levine & Stetson 1939). This antibody caused a severe transfusion reaction in a woman who, after delivery of a stillborn fetus, had received a transfusion of her husband's blood. Levine & Stetson (1939) recognized that their patient may have been immunized by a property in the blood or tissues of her fetus which it had inherited from the father.

The following year Wiener & Peters (1940) described antibodies of the same specificity in three patients who had suffered haemolytic episodes after transfusion of ABO compatible blood. These anti-Rh D antibodies reacted with red cells from about 85% of the populations tested (Wiener & Peters 1940). The D antigen was the first described and clinically the most important antigen of the now complex Rh blood group system (for review see Race et al 1948).

Structure of the D antigen

Depending on the Rh phenotype, between about 10 000 and 33 000 D antigen sites are distributed, apparently randomly, over the surface of D-positive human red cells (Rochna & Hughes-Jones 1965). Because of the small quantities of D antigen in the membrane and difficulties encountered in isolating it, knowledge of the structure of D is limited. However, Green (1972) showed that the D antigen is a protein which is dependent on phospholipid for its expression.

In 1982 Moore et al adsorbed IgG anti-Rh D antibodies onto ^{125}I labelled intact red cells before solubilizing the membranes with detergent and isolating the antibody-antigen complexes with Staphylococcus protein A. SDS polyacrylamide gel electrophoresis revealed that D was mostly associated with a component of 28 500 apparent molecular weight. Gahmberg (1982, 1983) showed that a surface exposed polypeptide of apparent molecular weight between 28 000 and 33 000 was immunoprecipitated from D-positive but not D-negative red cell membranes by anti-Rh D antibodies, and that this polypeptide is not glycosylated. Ridgwell et al (1983) found that Rh$_{null}$ cells, which are devoid of all Rh antigens, lack two extracellular thiol-group containing components of 32 000 and 34 000 apparent molecular weight. The former was immunoprecipitated by human anti-Rh D antibody and the latter by a murine monoclonal antibody which reacts with all red cells except those of the Rh$_{null}$ phenotype. Ridgwell et al (1983) suggest that the 32 000 component corresponds to the D polypeptide of Moore et al (1982) and of Gahmberg (1982) and that D is likely to be a polymorphism carried on the 'D' protein.

In 1984 both Gahmberg & Karhi (1984) and Ridgwell et al (1984) found that the D polypeptide appears to be linked to the red cell skeletal matrix, suggesting that this polypeptide may play a functional role in the maintenance of red cell shape and viability. This could explain the reduced in vivo survival and abnormal shape of Rh$_{null}$ cells, deficient in this protein. Controversially, Plapp and his colleagues (Evans et al 1983, Sinar et al 1984) have consistently argued that a D-active lipoprotein can be isolated from red cell membranes of individuals of both D-positive and D-negative phenotypes, the D antigen being expressed on the outer surface of the cells of phenotypes traditionally regarded as D-positive and on the inner surface of those regarded as D-negative.

D^u and the D mosaic

In 1946 Stratton described a variant of the D antigen called D^u which reacted with some anti-Rh D antibodies but not others. It was soon appreciated (Stratton & Renton 1948, Race et al 1948) that the strength of D^u varies from 'high grade', in which the cells are agglutinated by some anti-Rh D sera, to 'low grade' which can only be detected by the antiglobulin test and occasionally only by adsorption and elution (Yvart et al 1974). Although D^u is generally inherited as an allele of D, D^u phenotype may result from the position effect of a Cde gene complex in trans with a normal D (Ceppellini et al 1955).

As there appears to be a spectrum of D antigen strength from D to low grade D^u, it is unfortunate that there is no precise definition distinguishing D from D^u. A different weak form of D is associated with the infrequent Rh antigen Rh33 (Giles 1971). Some rare Rh D positive individuals may make alloanti-D antibodies. If the D antigen is pictured as a mosaic then a D positive individual whose red cells lack part of that mosaic may, if immunized, make antibody to the portion of the D antigen they lack. As cells of most D positive individuals carry the whole D mosaic, this antibody generally behaves as an anti-Rh D antibody.

Wiener & Unger (1962) recognized four components of the D antigen, Rh^{ABCD}. Tippett & Sanger (1962) analyzed results of cross-testing cells and sera of D positive individuals who had made anti-Rh D antibodies and classified these D antigens into six categories. Three of the categories have subsequently been subdivided. Tippett & Sanger's (1977) scheme is shown in Table 11.1. Category I red cells reacted with all anti-D antibodies except their own but their anti-D is too weak to give reliable results: hence Category I has been abandoned. Category VI cells have the least D as determined by anti-D made by D-negative and D-positive individuals.

Two of the sub-categories, IVa and Va, are identified by specific antibodies, anti-Goᵃ and anti-Dᵂ, respectively (Table 11.1). These antibodies allow for recognition of the presence of D^{IVa} or D^{Va} genes, even when a normal D allele is present in trans. Anti-Tar is another antibody to a private antigen which specifically recognises the product of a variant D gene usually found in a CDe complex (Lewis et al 1979). Recently, two Tar-positive (CD^Te/cde) individuals with anti-Rh D antibodies in their serum were described by Lomas et al (1986) who proposed that D^T should become category VII. Table 11.2 briefly summarizes the seven categories.

Variants of D^u exist in which part of the D mosaic is missing and anti-D antibodies may be made, but these have not been categorized.

Table 11.1 Interaction between cells and serum of people with D on their cells and anti-D in their serum. (From Tippett & Sanger 1977.)

Cells	Sera												Anti-		
	II	III			IV			V			VI		G	Goᵃ	Dᵂ
		a	b	c	a	a	b	a	b	c	i	ii			
II	−	+	+	+	+	+	w	+	+	w	+	+	+	−	−
IIIa	+	−	+	−	+	+	+	+	+	+	+	+	+	−	−
IIIb	+	−	−	−	+	+	+	w	+	+	+	+	−	−	−
IIIc	+	−	+	−	+	+	+	+	+	+	+	+	+	−	−
IVa	−	w	+	−	−	−	−	+	+	−	+	+	+	+	−
IVb	−	w	+	w	−	−	−	−	+	w	+	−	+	−	−
Va	+	−	+	−	+	w	+	−	w	−	+	−	+	−	+
Vb	+	−	+	−	+	−	−	−	−	−	−	−	+	−	−
Vc	+	−	+	−	w	−	w	−	−	−	+	−	+	−	−
VI	−	−	+	−	+	−	+	−	−	−	−	−	+	−	−

Table 11.2 Tippett & Sanger's classification for D+ people with anti-D in their serum.

Category	Haplotype	Race	Comments
I	–	–	abandoned
II	$CD^{II}e$	white	3 unrelated members
III	$cD^{III}e$	mostly black	3 subdivisions
IV	$cD^{IV}e$	mostly black	cells usually $Go(a+)$ 2 subdivisions
V	usually cD^Ve or CD^Ve	black or white	cells usually D^w+ 3 subdivisions
VI	$CD^{VI}e$, $cD^{VI}e$ or $cD^{VI}e$	mostly white	heterogeneous group
VII	$CD^{VII}e$	white	cells Tar $+$

Rh haemolytic disease of the newborn

Mollison (1983) defines haemolytic disease of the newborn (HDN) as, 'A condition in which the life span of the infant's red cells is shortened by the action of specific antibodies derived from the mother by placental transfer'. An affected fetus may die in utero or may be born alive suffering a variety of symptoms including jaundice, which may lead to kernicterus, anaemia and generalized oedema. The infant's red cells usually give a positive direct antiglobulin test (DAT) although this is not definitive of HDN; DAT positive red cells may survive normally in the circulation (Mollison 1983).

Before preventative treatment was discovered anti-Rh D antibody was responsible for the vast majority of cases of HDN. Levine et al (1941) reported that in 93% of cases investigated, HDN resulted from immunization of an Rh-negative mother by the Rh factor in the red cells of the fetus. Severity of the disease is extremely variable. Rarely is Rh HDN encountered in a first pregnancy and usually the first infant with the disease is affected less severely than subsequent affected infants (see Mollison 1983).

Prophylaxis for Rh haemolytic disease of the newborn

The first recognition of the D antigen and its possible involvement in HDN came with the discovery of anti-D in 1939 and within a period of about 40 years the disease has been markedly reduced in developed countries. Rh immunization seldom occurs in mothers of ABO incompatible babies (Nevanlinna 1956), presumably because fetal red cells spilling into the bloodstream of the mother are rapidly removed by maternal anti-A or anti-B. This led to the idea, by groups both in England and the USA (Clarke & McConnell 1972), that injection of anti-D into a D-negative mother of a D-positive baby, soon after delivery, may suppress primary immunization. At first, attempts to suppress D immunization in D-negative male volunteers, using IgM anti-D, failed (Finn 1961). However, no immunization occurred when D-positive cells were administered followed by IgG anti-D (Clarke et al 1963). Clinical trials in Britain and the USA showed that injection of IgG anti-D immediately after parturition prevented primary immunization to the D antigen in the majority of D-negative mothers resulting in no production of anti-D during the subsequent pregnancy (Combined study 1966, 1971).

There can be no doubt about the success of the Rh immunization prophylaxis programme although the mechanism of action of this suppression of the immune response to the Rh D antigen is still controversial. The non-specific clearance of the antibody-coated Rh D positive red cells from the circulation by binding to the splenic macrophages is suggested as an important mechanism since when Rh D negative, Kell negative volunteers were immunized with Rh D positive, Kell positive red cells the anti D immune response could be prevented by an immediate dose of anti Kell antibody (Woodrow et al 1975). Other data suggest more specific and complex mechanisms involving active suppression of the immune response perhaps by the anti idiotype network (Natvig et al 1976). This is supported by clinical data showing that although anti-D prophylactic therapy has led to a dramatic reduction in the incidence of immunization to the D antigen, no change has been seen in the incidence of immunization to other Rhesus antigens in women receiving anti-D post partum (Tovey 1986).

At the present time all D-negative women are given an injection of between 100 μg and 400 μg of anti-D immunoglobulin within 72 hours of giving birth to a D positive baby (see Mollison 1983). Also, all D-negative women are treated following abortion, amniocentesis or fetal manipulation. However, sensitization still occurs at the rate of 600–800 women per year in the UK (Urbaniak 1985). This is usually due to sensitization occurring during the pregnancy, and for this reason in some countries an injection of anti-D immunoglobulin is given to all D negative women antenatally (at 28 and 34 weeks gestation) to protect against immunization during the course of their pregnancy (Bowman 1984). This practice has recently been recommended in the UK for Rh D negative mothers in their first pregnancy (Drug & Therapeutics Bulletin 1985).

Anti-D immunoglobulin is obtained from deliberately immunized or boosted volunteers and is an expensive and valuable resource involving inconvenience and some hazard to the donor. As demand for this material increases it would be advantageous to be able to manufacture unlimited quantities in vitro. Development of the methods of production of monoclonal anti-D clearly opens up the possibility of achieving this aim.

MONOCLONAL ANTIBODIES

In 1975 Köhler and Milstein described the use of cell fusion between cells of a mouse myeloma cell line and spleen cells from immunized mice to

Table 11.3   Mouse monoclonal antibodies to red cell antigens.

Antigen	Reference
A1	Voak et al 1982
B	Voak et al 1982
H	Doinel et al 1983
M	Bigbee et al 1983
N	Fraser et al 1982
Le^a	Young et al 1983
Le^b	Brockaus et al 1981

produce hybrids which secrete antibodies of a predetermined specificity (Köhler & Milstein 1975). Because of their origin from a single cell the antibodies produced by these hybrids are monoclonal and therefore show remarkable antigenic specificity (for review see Beverley 1980). Prior to this time specific antisera obtained from human subjects or raised in laboratory animals were used as tools for routine and research assay systems as well as for passive immunization in humans. These polyclonal antisera have certain disadvantages, such as a limited supply and non-specificity, which monoclonal reagents can overcome. Thus, as a result of their clonal origin monoclonal antibodies (MAbs) are exquisitely specific reagents, and their in vitro production allows for an unlimited supply of standard reagents. Within haematology, MAbs have allowed the delineation of cell markers associated with the phylogeny and ontogeny of the haematological cell types and have aided the classification and diagnosis of the leukaemias (Linch & Griffin 1986). Blood transfusion laboratories have gained specific red blood cell typing reagents (Table 11.3). Early criticisms that monoclonal reagents may be too specific to act as useful red cell typing reagents have been offset by the pooling of antibodies of different specificities.

Unfortunately, despite much effort, no mouse or rat MAbs have yet been reported which are specific for the Rh D antigen. This finding probably reflects the fact that despite its restriction to human red cells the Rh D antigen is non immunogenic in laboratory animals.

Human monoclonal antibodies

Despite the tremendous clinical potential of rodent MAbs there are some situations in which the xenogeneic nature of these molecules is a disadvantage. These include their in vivo use in humans for prophylaxis, diagnosis and therapy, where human MAbs would provide an unlimited supply of material. The use of MAbs would be safer than the material purified from human serum which is used at present and which may carry the risk of contamination with pathogens such as hepatitis B virus or human immunodeficiency virus (HIV). Preliminary studies in this area using mouse MAbs have indicated that an antibody response to the xenogeneic immunoglobulin molecule may develop, and that subsequent therapy is ineffective (Schroff

Table 11.4   The uses of human monoclonal antibodies.

Use	Example
In vivo therapy in man	– Anti-Rh D in HDN prophylaxis – Antimicrobial agents – Cancer therapy and imaging – Anti-lymphocyte globulin for immunosuppression – Anti-poison agents in drug toxicity
Production of reagents recognising epitopes identified by the human immune response	– Anti-HLA MAbs for typing reagents – Antibacterial MAbs to identify strain and subtype differences
Study of the human immune repertoire to specific antigens	– Infectious agents – Tumour cells
Study of the autoimmune response	– Systemic lupus erythematosis – Rheumatoid arthritis – Autoimmune haemolytic anaemia
Production of MAbs to antigens non-immunogenic in rodents	– Rh D

et al 1985). Thus their application may be limited to one dose or one course of treatment. In this situation MAbs obtained from humans would be advantageous as they would in all probability be less immunogenic. Other situations in which human MAbs would be useful are shown in Table 11.4.

The Rh D antigen has been a popular choice for attempts to make human MAbs because of its importance in vivo use in the prevention of HDN, where supplies of antibody purified from human serum may be in short supply. Furthermore, in the absence of a rodent MAb human reagents could also be used for routine red cell typing.

At present three methods are available for human MAb production:
1. Cell fusion (for review see Kozbor & Croce 1985).
2. Epstein-Barr virus (EBV) immortalisation (for review see Crawford 1985).
3. EBV immortalisation followed by cell fusion (for review see Roder et al 1985).
Each of these methods has been used successfully to produce MAbs to the Rh D antigen.

Cell fusion

The cell hybridisation method developed by Köhler & Milstein (1975) for rodent cells has not proved as effective when used in the human system. Two main factors appear to be responsible for this: (a) a lack of suitable cell lines for fusion and (b) a lack of adequate numbers of specifically activated B cells.

Initially it was assumed that human myeloma cell lines would form the best fusion partners because of their innate ability to secrete high levels of immunoglobulin. However, great difficulty has been experienced in adapting these cells to long term growth in culture. Only a few such cell lines exist and these grow slowly and have proved to be very inefficient at fusing with human B cells. To overcome this problem, faster growing EB virus-transformed lymphoblastoid cell lines have been used as fusion partners. However, here again the rate of fusion is very low, and this now appears to be a property of human lymphoid cells in general. For this reason the fusion of human cells to mouse myeloma cell lines has been used in some instances. The disadvantage in such fusions appears to be the preferential loss of human chromosomes from the resultant hybrids. Human chromosome 2 which carries the K-immunoglobulin light chain gene is lost preferentially and other disturbances of gene expression may also cause loss of antibody production. Finally, heteromyelomas, that is mouse-human myeloma hybrids, have been used as fusion partners (Teng et al 1983) in an effort to overcome these problems. Theoretically, such cell lines would retain the greater fusion capability of the mouse myeloma line and the presence of human chromosomes would provide stability to the resultant hybrids. The frequency of fusion reported here is greater than with human myeloma cells, however the technique remains to be assessed in detail. Using this system Bron et al (1984) have made several MAbs including one to Rh D antigen.

In the mouse system, spleen B cells are used for fusion following in vivo stimulation with antigen. This cell fusion is facilitated by having both the fusion partners as actively dividing cells in the G1 phase of the cell cycle. In humans, peripheral blood is usually the only source of B cells available, and here activated B cells in the appropriate stage of cell cycle are not present unless the subject has been recently immunized. This constitutes a major disadvantage which has only been partially overcome by in vitro expansion of sensitized B cells with polyclonal activators. Pokeweed mitogen and *Staphylococcus aureus* Cowan A have been used without much success (Teng et al 1986). EBV transformation prior to hybridisation is commonly used to expand the antigen specific population (see below), and in vitro sensitization of B cells with antigen has produced some antibody-secreting clones (Crawford et al 1983).

Epstein-Barr virus (EBV) immortalisation

EBV is a human lymphotrophic herpes virus which is aetiologically associated with a wide range of clinical syndromes – acute and chronic infectious mononucleoses, African Burkitt's Lymphoma, undifferentiated nasopharyngeal carcinoma and 'lymphoma' in the immunosuppressed. Most people become infected by the virus in childhood without clinical manifestations and acquire circulating antibodies to viral antigens (for review see Crawford & Edwards 1986).

In vitro, EBV infects B cells, (Pattengale et al 1973), polyclonally activates them (Rosen et al 1977) and immortalizes them into continuously growing lymphoblastoid cell lines. The particular affinity of EBV to B cells is due to the presence, on the B cell surface, of the CR2 receptor which also acts as the receptor for EBV (Frade et al 1985). Once EBV has infected a B cell a series of events occur leading to the activation of the cell. The EBV-associated nuclear antigen complex (EBNA) can be detected within 12 hours and constitutes the hallmark of EBV infection. This is followed by blastogenesis at 24 hours and cellular DNA synthesis by 36 hours leading to cell proliferation and immortalisation (Fig. 11.1). These cells will continue to proliferate indefinitely in culture as B lymphoblastoid cell lines.

EBV not only immortalizes B cells but also activates them to secrete immunoglobulin in a T cell independent manner (Rosen et al 1977). Immunoglobulin can be detected in the culture supernatant of B cells 4–5 days post-infection and remains at high levels (10–30 μg/ml) for 4–8 weeks. Thereafter, without cloning, it declines and stabilizes to low levels (0.1–10 μg/ml); IgM usually predominates.

Although the vast majority of circulating B cells express CR2 receptors and bind EB virus particles to their surface, only a small percentage of these cells actually become polyclonally activated and/or immortalized (Fig. 11.1). Furthermore, whereas most immortalized cells synthesise immunoglobulin, there is an identifiable population of cells which become activated by the virus to secrete immunoglobulin but are short lived, surviving only the first 4–6 weeks of the culture period. These observations suggest that although the events of activation and immortalization share the initial infection step, thereafter their pathways diverge; however the cellular events involved in these processes are uncertain.

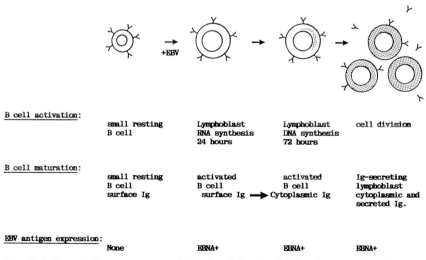

B cell activation:				
	small resting B cell	Lymphoblast RNA synthesis 24 hours	Lymphoblast DNA synthesis 72 hours	cell division

B cell maturation:				
	small resting B cell surface Ig	activated B cell surface Ig ➝ Cytoplasmic Ig	activated B cell	Ig-secreting lymphoblast cytoplasmic and secreted Ig.

EBV antigen expression:				
	None	EBNA+	EBNA+	EBNA+

Fig. 11.1 The cellular consequences of EB virus infection of B lymphocytes. Y = Ig molecule. ⊞ = cytoplasmic Ig.

The properties of polyclonal activation and immortalization of B cells by EBV have been exploited for making human MAbs in vitro. This was first reported by Steinitz et al (1977) and thereafter many MAbs have been made using this technique, including several to the Rh D antigen (Crawford et al 1983a, Bron et al 1984, Doyle et al 1985, Thompson et al 1986).

In spite of the apparent suitability of EBV as an agent for making human MAb producing cell lines, certain technical problems remain to be solved. Specific antibody production from such cell lines may be short lived and the reason for this is unclear. One of the causes may be the very low numbers of specific antibody-producing B cells in the circulation. Thus EBV infection of a non-specific B cell population leads to activation and immortalization of non-antigen specific B cells which are likely to overgrow the small number of specific B cells if cloning is not carried out early in the culture period. It may be that the specific immunoglobulin secreting B cells are intrinsically short lived (Crawford 1985), which may reflect a failure in immortalization events following infection and activation; lose their receptor for B cell growth factors (Melamed et al 1985) or have stricter nutritional requirements than the non-antibody-producing cells (Crawford 1985). Finally, the cloning efficiency of EBV transfromed B cells is not very high (1–3% at 1 cell/well) (Crawford 1985) which makes it difficult to isolate specific antibody-producing clones from a polyclonal cell line.

EBV Immortalization followed by cell fusion

The methods of cell fusion and EBV immortalization alone have not proved very effective in giving stable antibody-producing clones, but a combination of the two is showing some promise. B cells producing specific immunoglobulin are expanded in vitro by EBV immortalization and before antibody production is lost the specific antibody-producing cells are fused to a suitable fusion partner. Hybrids are then grown in selective medium to which ouabain is added. Mouse cells are naturally about 10 000 times more resistant to ouabain than human cells making this a suitable drug for selectively killing the unfused cells of the human B cell line. However, if a human fusion partner is used it has to be previously selected for ouabain resistance. Several stable MAbs have been made by this technique and include those to blood group A antigen (Foung et al 1986), Rh D antigen (Thompson et al 1986) and RhG antigen (Foung et al 1986). Reports of fairly high frequencies of fusion, with high levels of antibody secretion, which appears to be stable, make this method worth further study.

Efficiency of human monoclonal antibody production

All the methods described for the production of human MAbs are appreciably less efficient than the classical method of cell fusion for the production of mouse or rat MAbs. Efforts to increase this efficiency have included:

a. Appropriate donor selection
b. Enrichment for specific antibody-producing cells and
c. Increased cloning efficiency.

These criteria have been applied to the production of human MAbs to the Rh D antigen with a fair amount of success.

Donor selection

In order to obtain specific antibody-producing cells from peripheral blood it is advantageous to prime the donors with antigen, since it has been shown that following secondary tetanus toxoid immunization antibody-producing cells only circulate for six weeks peaking at two weeks (Kozbor & Roder 1981). Such cells from Rh D primed donors may be obtained from blood transfusion centres where a programme of immunization of Rh negative volunteers is being undertaken for the production of polyclonal Rh D antibody. Another source is Rh D negative mothers immunized by pregnancy. In the former case multiply immunized indiviudals are preferable since the primary antibody response to the D antigen is often weak and delayed (Mollison 1983). Some controversy exists as to the type of B cells susceptible to infection and immortalization by EBV, since it was initially reported that small resting memory B cells are the target cells for immortalization (Aman et al 1984). However, a more recent report suggests that large activated cells may also be susceptible (Chan et al 1986). If the latter were the case, cells obtained early after immunization would be preferable; however, if the former case applies then success would be more likely if cells were harvested after the initial activated cell reaction had subsided.

Enrichment of specific antibody producing cells

The enrichment of specific antibody-producing cells has been undertaken in a variety of ways and leads to an increased efficiency of production of specific antibody-producing cell lines. Several methods have been used successfully including: rosetting with specific antigen-coated red blood cells (Steinitz et al 1977, 1979, 1982, Crawford et al 1983a), panning onto antigen coated plates (Winger et al 1983) and separating on the flourescence activated cell sorter (FACS) after binding of fluorescence labelled antigen to the surface of antigen specific cells (Kozbor & Roder 1981). For red cell antigens rosetting is the method of choice since RBCs naturally expressing the appropriate antigen can be used. Enrichment of anti-Rh D-producing B cells has been successful using Rh positive RBCs (Table 11.5).

In vitro stimulation with specific antigen has also been achieved. Primary in vitro sensitization has been reported using a variety of antigens (Winger

Table 11.5a   Published human monoclonal antibodies to RhD. Methods used in production.

Reference	Donor	Immort.	Method of Enrichment	Cloning
Koskimies 1980	Immunised male volunteer boosted 1 month before bleeding	EBV infection	Rosetting with A Rh+ RBCs before and after infection	None
Boylston et al 1980	Female sensitised during pregnancy. Bled 8 days after boosting	EBV infection	Rosetting with ORh+ RBCs after infection	None
Crawford et al 1983a	Immunised male volunteer boosted 7 days before bleeding	EBV infection	Rosetting with -D- RBCs before infection	LD*
Bron et al 1984	Female sensitised during pregnancy. Bled 2 weeks after delivery	EBV + cell fusion	Rosetting with ORh+ RBCs after infection	LD
Doyle et al 1985	Female sensitised during pregnancy. Boosted 8 days before bleeding	EBV infection	Rosetting with ORh+ RBCs after infection	LD
Thompson et al 1986	Immunised male volunteer boosted 7 weeks before bleeding	EBV + cell fusion	None	LD
Broly & Huart 1986	NS	EBV infection	NS	LD
Paire et al 1986	Immunised donors	EBV infection	Rosetting after infection	LD

* LD = limiting dilution
NS = not stated

et al 1983) and a human MAb to the influenza virus has been produced by in vitro secondary stimulation of lymphocytes following natural primary infection (Crawford et al 1983b).

Increased cloning efficiency

Overgrowth of specific antibody-producing B cells by non producers in the culture, despite enrichment procedures, necessitates early and efficient cloning. For this an appropriate feeder cell layer is essential and in our hands, irradiated allogeneic peripheral blood mononuclear cells have been shown to give the highest cloning efficiency. However, there is marked variation in ability to support clonal growth between different cell types as well as between individual donors. The reason for this is unknown but may be related to differences in growth factor production.

Table 11.5b   Published human monoclonal antibodies to Rh D. Characterization of anti RhD antibody.

Reference	Designation	Antibody Type	Antibody Levels	Stability
Koskimies 1980	KS-P	IgG3K	2–8 µg/ml	12 months
Boylston et al 1980	NS*	IgM	2–5 µg/ml	Specific activity lost after 12–14 weeks
Crawford et al 1983a	UCH D4	IgG1K	10–20 µg/ml	Stable >4 years
Bron et al 1984	D4–B2 E10–C1	IgG3	12–20 µg/ml	Stable >8 months
Doyle et al 1985	FC3	IgG1	20 µg/ml	Stable >10 months
Thompson et al 1986	MAD2 GAD2	IgM IgG	25–50 µg/ml	Stable >10 months
Broly & Huart 1986	65	IgM	NS	NS
Paire et al 1986	CO 118.8 CO 117.12	IgG1λ IgG1λ	12 µ/ml 5 µ/ml	2 years 2 years

* NS = not stated

Monoclonal antibodies to the Rh D antigen

Despite the overall success in the production of rodent monoclonal antibodies to specified antigens no such monoclonal reagents have been produced to the Rh D antigens. This may be because these antigens, which only occur on human red cells, are not recognized by the mouse or rat immune system. Fortunately in this instance the human system has proved more successful, and several MAbs have been reported (Crawford et al 1983a, Doyle et al 1985, Bron et al 1984, Thompson et al 1986). The characteristics of these MAbs and their methods of production are shown in Table 11.5. This success may reflect the accessability of recently primed donors which have been the source of B cells in most cases. Specific antibody-producing B cells may be separated by rosetting with Rh positive RBCs. We have used red cells of the -D- phenotype because these possess more Rh D antigenic sites per cell (200 000 as compared to 20–30 000) and form more stable rosettes. Once separated the specific B cells have been infected with EBV and cultured. We have had increased success by plating low cell numbers initially. This necessitates a feeder layer to maintain cell growth, but minimizes the overgrowth of non-antibody secreting cells. After 2–3 weeks in culture the supernatant medium is screened for antibody production using papain-treated Rh positive RBCs, and positive cultures cloned by limiting dilution. Many such clones are successfully growing and producing antibody after several years in culture. Others have been stabilized by fusion to mouse myeloma cells.

Most of the antibodies produced are IgG with two IgM and one IgA (Table 11.5). This is unusual since EBV has a predilection for IgM producing cells, but may reflect the multimmunised status of the donors.

We have compared a panel of six of these antibodies (Table 11.6) for their reactivity against D positive and negative cells by the saline, papain and antiglobulin methods (Table 11.7) and against a panel of cells of various D categories (Table 11.8). Only one antibody (No. 6) directly agglutinated D+ cells. All reacted with papain treated D+ RBCs and in the antiglobulin test using anti-human globulin; one antibody (No. 2) reacted only weakly. However, because of the lack of standardization of concentration of antibody in the culture supernatant provided, titres and quantities of antibody cannot be directly compared between antibodies from different batches. Generally these antibodies should make good typing reagents for laboratory use.

The reactivity of the monoclonals with the D categories shows an overall similar pattern. In some categories the variation in strength reflects the variation in D expression observed with polyclonal reagents. For example, only some samples with D^{Va} antigens are agglutinated by antibody No. 6,

Table 11.6 Monoclonal antibodies to the Rh D antigen.

No.	MAbs	Reference	IMMUNOGLOBULIN	
			Class	Sub-class
1	Co 8.8.A	Paire et al 1986 Immunology letters	G	
2	CD6	Kumpel et al (in press)	G	G3
3	FC3	Doyle et al 1985	G	G1
4	UCHD4	Crawford 1983a	G	G1
5	K5	Crawford, unpublished data	A	—
6	85–12	Okubo (personal communication)*	G	G1

* Y Okubo, Osaka Red Cross, Osaka, Japan

Table 11.7 Titre of MAbs with Rhesus D Negative (Cde/cde) and D Positive (cDe/cde) red blood cells.

Test	Genotype of RBC	monoclonal antibodies*					
		1	2	3	4	5	6
Saline	cDe/cde	—	—	—	—	—	256
	Cde/cde	—	—	—	—	—	—
Papain-treated RBC	cDe/cde	256	16	256	256	64	256
	Cde/cde	—	—	—	—	—	—
Anti-globulin Test	cDe/cde	+	+	+	+	+	+
	Cde/cde	—	—	—	—	—	—

* Names shown in Table 11.6

Table 11.8 Reaction of MAbs with Rhesus D categories.

Rh genotype	IIIa cDe/cde	IIIc CDe/cde	IVa cDe/cde	IVb CDe/cde	Va cDe/cde	Va CDe/cde	Va cDE/cde	VI cDE/cde	VI CDe/cde	VII* CDe/cde	Rh:33 C(D)(e)/cde	$cD^{u}e$/cde
No. of RBC samples	1	1	5	1	1	1	1	1	1	2	2	1
Test — Mabs** 1	+	+	+	+	+	+	+	−	−	+	−	−
2	+	+	+	+	+	+	+	−	−	+	−	+
3	+	+	+	+	+	+	+	NT	−	+	−	+
Papain-treated cells 4	+	+	+	−	+	+	+	−	−	+	−	+
5	+	+	+	NT	+	+	+	−	−	+	−	NT
6	+	+	+	+	−	−	+	−	−	+/−	−	−
saline 6	+	w	+	w	−	−	+	−	−	w/−	−	−

* VII = Tar+

NT = Not tested

Variations within a category reflects the variation of D expression

** Names shown in Table 11.6

w = Weakly positive

although all react when papain treated. Confirmation of negative results should be attempted by adsorption and elution tests.

If, as has been previously suggested, the D antigen is a mosaic structure with several antigenic sites, some of which are absent on D category RBCs, more variability in reactivity with this RBC panel would have been expected from six MAbs. None of the MAbs reacted with category VI cells by the methods used. Crawford et al (1984) found that antibody No. 4 reacted weakly with category VI samples by an antiglobulin technique. This anomaly may indicate variability in antibody concentration between different batches or the difference in sensitivity of different methods. The failure of IVb cells to react with antibody No. 4 suggests that D^{IVb} differs from D^{IVa} antigen. Tests with further examples of monoclonal anti-D and biochemical studies should help to elucidate the complexities of the D mosaic. The reaction pattern of MAbs made using B cells isolated from individuals with D category RBCs would also be of interest.

IN VIVO USE OF HUMAN ANTI RH-D MONOCLONAL ANTIBODIES

Since anti-Rh D for the prophylaxis of HDN is in short supply it seems reasonable to investigate the use of human monoclonal antibodies for this purpose. If effective this would form an unlimited supply of a safer, standardized therapeutic product. Although the exact mechanism of action of prophylactic antibody is not clear, it probably involves the coating of Rh positive cells in the circulation with specific antibody, and the subsequent removal of these cells by mononuclear phagocytes in the spleen. This mechanism depends on the Fc portion of the antibody molecule binding to Fc receptors on mononuclear phagocytes, which is mainly a property of human immunoglobulin subclasses of IgG1 and IgG3. This mechanism may be enhanced by complement components binding to the immunoglobulin Fc and to complement receptors on the phagocyte surface, although anti-D antibodies are very rarely complement-binding. The property of phagocyte binding can be tested for in vitro by incubating antibody-coated Rh positive RBCs with purified blood monocytes, and counting the proportion of ingested cells. This has been shown to be negative with our anti-D human MAb UCH D4 (antibody No. 4 in Table 11.6).

Purification of antibody for in vivo use

Culture supernatant medium from EBV genome-containing lymphoblastoid cell lines contains cellular and viral DNA as well as infectious EB virus particles. Despite the fact that EBV is associated with the geographically restricted malignant human tumours, African Burkitt's lymphoma and anaplastic nasopharyngeal carcinoma, as well as 'lymphomas' in immunosuppressed patients, we have argued that administration of MAb purified from this source to normal individuals is a safe procedure (Crawford et al 1983c). This is based on the facts that:

1. The virus is ubiquitous – over 90% of adults are seropositive for the virus, and continue to harbour the virus in a few circulating B lymphocytes, with intermittent secretion into the saliva.

2. Blood and blood products from seropositive individuals must contain EB viral DNA, and are apparently harmless when given to sero-negative individuals. In particular, there is no reported increased incidence of lymphoma following blood transfusion, although transfusion mononucleosis due to EBV has been reported following transfusion of large quantities of fresh blood (Gerber et al 1969).

3. Antibodies for injection are prepared by cold ethanol precipitation from pooled human serum which is not screened for antibodies to EBV antigens. These products are regularly given to hypogammaglobulinaemic or agammaglobulinaemic patients with no apparent ill effect.

4. A method for the purification of antibody from culture supernatant material has been tested in spiking experiments and found to remove both DNA and infectious EB virus to the limits of detection. Thus in six experiments where 1 mg/ml of DNA was added to UCH D4 supernatant, less than 0.01 μg/ml (the lower limit of sensitivity of the method used) was detected after purification. Similarly, concentrated, infectious EB virus added to the culture supernatant could not be detected in the purified product when assayed by transformation of cord blood mononuclear cells. From these experiments it can be calculated that each 1 ml dose of purified UCH D4 antibody (containing 150 μg of anti-D) would contain less than one EBV genome equivalent of DNA (Crawford et al 1984). These findings are similar to those of Finter and Fantes (1980) for the purification of interferon from the EBV genome-containing Burkitt's lymphoma cell line, Namalva (Finter & Fantes 1980). This product is already on the market and is apparently without side effects attributable to EBV.

The purification steps used by us for the preparation of UCH D4 antibody for in vivo use are as follows:

1. Filter culture supernatant medium through a 0.22 μm followed by a 0.1 μm filter to remove cells, cell debris and virus particles.
2. Treat with DNase for one hour at 37°C to digest residual DNA.
3. Pass down an anti IgG column to bind specific antibody and allow passage of contaminants.
4. Wash column in borate buffer and elute antibody using 0.5% acetic acid.
5. Dialyse antibody against normal saline, and concentrate.
6. Filter through 0.22 μm filter to sterilize.
7. Pyrogen test in rabbits.

The procedure was undertaken in pyrogen-free glassware and the antibody stored in 1 ml ampoules at −20°C.

In vivo experiments

In order to test UCH D4 in vivo for its ability to remove Rh positive cells from the circulation and prevent an immune response to these cells two experimental designs were used. In the first experiment a Rh-positive male volunteer who was positive for antibodies to EBV antigens and negative for hepatitis B surface antigen (HBs) was chosen. RBCs from the volunteer were labelled with ^{51}Cr, coated with 1 ml (150 μg/ml) of purified UCH D4 antibody with a titre in the anti-immunoglobulin test of 1 : 500 and re-injected. Counts were taken over the heart, liver and spleen for one hour and then for 10 minutes daily for three days. A routine RBC survival analysis was carried out on the labelled cells.

In the second experiment a Rh negative male volunteer who was sero-positive for antibodies to EB viral antigens and HBs antigen negative was chosen. He was given an intramuscular 1 ml dose of purified UCHD4 containing 150 μg of antibody. Three days later, when anti-D could be detected in his serum, 1 ml of packed, ^{51}Cr labelled, Rh positive RBC was injected intravenously. These cells had been matched to those of the volunteer for all RBC antigens except Rh D. Again, monitoring was carried out for one hour over the heart, liver and spleen, and then for 10 minutes daily for three days. A routine RBC survival analysis was also carried out.

In each case the survival of the injected RBCs in the circulation was normal (Fig. 11.2), with no sequestration noted in the liver or spleen. These results indicate that UCHD4, although an IgG1 antibody, is non-opsonising and therefore does not cause removal of coated RBCs from the circulation. This has confirmed the in vitro finding of the inability of the antibody to cause phagocytosis of coated RBCs.

Although this result is disappointing, it does not mean that UCHD4 does not protect against immunization with the D antigen since antibody coating of cells in the circulation may be sufficient. Follow up of the Rh negative volunteer is at present in progress.

Conclusions and future perspectives

The production of monoclonal antibodies to the Rh D antigen has been fairly successful over recent years, and several such antibodies have been reported, all of which are of human origin. These antibodies appear to have a very similar and comprehensive reactivity with a panel of D^u and D category red cells, and they should therefore make good red cell typing reagents for routine laboratory use. The change from polyclonal to mono-clonal reagents for red cell typing should occur universally in the next 2–3 years and will thus release a large volume of polyclonal antibody which can then be rechannelled for in vivo therapy. This should go some way to relieve the acute shortage of anti-D at present available for prophylaxis therapy in a country such as the UK, and allow the implementation of an

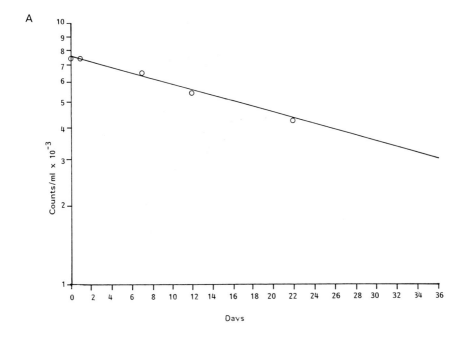

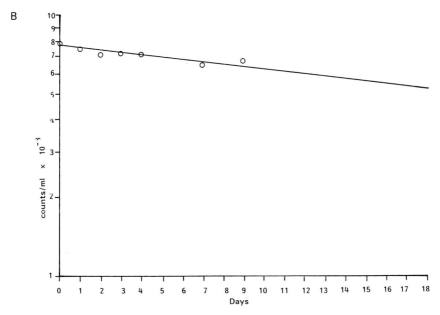

Fig. 11.2 Red cell survival in (a) human Rh positive volunteer receiving UCH D4 antibody-coated, ^{51}Cr-labelled, Rh positive RBCs (b) human Rh negative volunteer receiving ^{51}Cr-labelled, Rh positive RBCs three days after an intramuscular injection of UCH D4 antibody. The red cell survival is plotted as (a) 28.3 days, (b) 26 days, normal range 25–30 days. (Semi-log scale.)

antenatal prophylaxis programme. However, there is little doubt that in the long term monoclonal reagents produced in vitro will give an unlimited supply of a safer, standardized product for this purpose. For this to occur within a 5–10 year time span large scale trials of these antibodies must be planned along the lines of the preliminary testing described above. Because of the inherent variability in the immune response to the D antigen noted between individual volunteers large numbers would be needed to complete such trials. Furthermore, it is most likely that the best protection will be afforded by a cocktail of monoclonal antibodies of differing IgG subclass rather than individual reagents, and determining the ideal mix will necessitate more volunteers. Thus there is an urgent need for a multicentre trial to be undertaken by the large transfusion centres where Rh D immunization of volunteers is already a routine procedure for the production of polyclonal anti-D antibody.

Acknowledgements

The authors thank Dr P. Tippett and Ms C. Lomas for help with in vitro testing of the antibody panel and Dr M. Contreras, Ms P Teesdale, Dr M. Short, Ms G. Clarke and Ms M. Barlow for help with in vivo testing of UCHD4. We also thank Dr P. Tippett, Professor P. Mollison, and Dr M. Contreras for helpful discussions, and Ms E. Bashford for typing the manuscript.

REFERENCES

Aman P, Ehlin-Henriksson B, Klein G 1984 Epstein-Barr virus susceptibility of normal human B lymphocyte populations. Journal of Experimental Medicine 159: 208–220

Beverley P C L 1980 Production and use of monoclonal antibodies in transplantation immunology (Proceedings of the Eleventh International Course on Transplantation and Clinical Immunology) Excerpta Medica, Amsterdam, p 87–945

Bigbee W L, Vandervlaan M, Fong S S N, Jensen R H 1983 Monoclonal antibodies specific for the M- and N- forms of human glycophorin A. Molecular Immunology 20: 1353–1362

Bowman J M 1984 Controversies in Rh prophylaxis. In: Garratty (ed) Hemolytic disease of the newborn. American Association of Blood Banks, Arlington, VA

Boylston A W, Gardner B, Anderson L R, Hughes-Jones N C 1980 Production of human IgM anti-D in tissue culture by EB virus-transformed lymphocytes. Scandinavian Journal of Immunology 12: 355–358

Broly H, Huart J J 1986 Development d'un novelle technique simplified du groupafe Rhésus. Revere française des laboratoires. 147: 67–72

Brockhaus M, Mangani J L, Blaszezyk M et al 1981 Monoclonal antibodies directed against the human Le^b blood group antigen. Journal of Biological Chemistry 256: 13223–13225

Bron D, Feinberg M B, Teng N N H, Kaplan H S 1984 Production of human monoclonal IgG antibodies against Rhesus (D) antigen. Proceedings of the National Academy of Science USA 81: 3214–3217

Chan M A, Stein L D, Dosch H-M, Sigal N H 1986 Heterogeneity of EBV-transformable human B lymphocyte populations. Journal of Immunology 136: 106–112

Ceppellini R, Dunn L C, Turri M 1955 An interaction between alleles at the Rh locus in man which weakens the reactivity of the Rh$_o$ factor (D^u). Proceedings of the National Academy of Science, USA 41: 283–288

Clarke C A, McConell R B 1972 Prevention of Rh hemolytic disease. American Lecture Series. C C Thomas, Springfield, Illinois

Clarke C A, Donohoe W T A, McConnell R B et al 1963 Further experimental studies on the prevention of Rh haemolytic disease. British Medical Journal 1: 979–984

Crawford D H 1985 Production of human monoclonal antibodies using Epstein-Barr virus. Human hybridomas and monoclonal antibodies. Plenum Press, New York

Crawford D H, Edwards J M B 1986 The Epstein-Barr virus. Principles and practice of clinical virology. John Wiley, New York, p 111–122 1987

Crawford D H, Barlow M J, Harrison J F, Winger L, Huehns E R 1983a Production of human monoclonal antibody to Rhesus D antigen. Lancet 1: 386–388

Crawford D H, Callard R E, Muggeridge M I, Mitchell D M, Zanders E D, Beverley P C L 1983b Production of human monoclonal antibody to X31 influenza virus nucleoprotein. Journal of General Virology 64: 697–700

Crawford D H, Huehns E R, Epstein M A 1983c Therapeutic use of human monoclonal antibodies. Lancet 1:1040

Crawford D H, McDougall C J, Mulholland N, Zanders E D, Tippett P, Huehns E R 1984 Further characterisation of a human monoclonal antibody to the Rhesus D antigen produced in vitro. Behring Institute Mitteilungen 74: 55–60

Doinel C, Edelman L, Rouger P et al 1983 A murine monoclonal antibody against blood group H type-1 and type-2 structures. Immunology 50: 215–212

Doyle A, Jones T J, Bidwell J L, Bradley B A 1985 In vitro development of human monoclonal antibody-secreting plasmacytomas. Human Immunology 13: 199–209

Drug and Therapeutics Bulletin Editorial 1985 Anti-D immunologloglobulin prophylaxis – are we doing enough? Drug and Therapeutics Bulletin 23: 93–95

Evans J P, Brown P J, Sinor L T, Tilzer L L, Beck M, Plapp F V 1983 Detection of an antigen on the inner surface of Rh negative erythrocytes which binds anti-D IgG. Molecular Immunology 20: 529–536

Finn R, Clarke C A, Donohoe W T A, et al 1961 Experimental stuides on the prevention of Rh haemolytic disease. British Medical Journal 1: 1486–1490

Finter N B, Fantes K H 1980 The purity and safety of interferons prepared for clinical use: the case for lymphoblastoid interferon. In: Gresser I (ed) Interferon 2. Academic Press, New York

Foung S K H, Perkins S, Arvin A, et al 1986 Human hybridomas and monoclonal antibodies. Plenum Press, New York

Frade R, Barel M, Ehlin-Henrikkson B, Klein G 1985 gp 140, The C3d receptor of human B lymphocytes, is also the Epstein-Barr virus receptor. Proceedings of the National Academy of Science USA 82: 1490–1493

Fraser R H, Munro A C, Williamson A R et al 1982 Mouse monoclonal anti-N. I. Production and serological characterisation. Journal of Immunogenetics 9: 295–301

Gahmberg C G 1983 Molecular characterization of the human red cell $Rh_o(D)$ antigen. European molecular Biology Organization Journal 2: 223–227

Gahmberg C G 1982 Molecular identification of the human $Rh_o(D)$ antigen. Federation of European Biochemichal Societies Letters 140: 93–97

Gahmberg C G, Karhi K K 1984 Association of $Rh_o(D)$-polypeptides with the membrane skeleton in $Rh_o(D)$-positive human red cells. Journal of Immunology b133: 334–337

Gerber P, Walsh J H, Rosenblum E N, Purcell R H 1969 Association of EB-virus infection with the post-perfusion syndrome. Lancet 1: 593–596

Giles G, Crossland J D, Haggas W K, Longster G 1971 An Rh gene complex which results in a 'new' antigen detectable by a specific antibody, anti-Rh33. Vox Sanguinis 21: 289–301

Green F A 1972 Erythrocyte membrane lipids and Rh antigen activity. Journal of Biological Chemistry 247: 881–887

Köhler G, Milstein C 1975 Continuous cultures of fused cells secreting antibody of predefined specificity. Nature 256:496

Koskimies S 1980 Human lymphoblastoid cell live producing specific antibody against Rh-antigen D. Scandinavian Journal of Immunology 11: 73–77

Kozbor D, Croce C M 1985 Human hybridomas and monoclonal antibodies. Plenum Press, New York

Kozbor D, Roder J C 1981 Requirements for the establishment of high titered human monoclonal antibodies against tetanus toxoid using the Epstein-Barr virus technique. Journal of Immunology 127: 1275–1280

Levine P, Burnham L, Katzin E M, vogel P 1941 The role of isoimmunization in the pathogenesis of erythroblastosis fetalis. American Journal of Obstetrics and Gynaecology 42: 925–937

Levine P, Stetson R E 1939 An unusual case of intragroup agglutination. Journal of the American Medical Association 113: 126–127

Lewis M, Kaita H, Allerdice P W, Bartlett S, Squires W G, Huntsman R G 1979 Assignment of the red cell antigen Targett (Rh40), to the Rh blood group system. American Journal of Human Genetics 31: 630–633

Linch D C, Griffin J D 1986 Monoclonal antibodies reactive with myeloid associated antigens. Methods in Haematology No. 13. Monoclonal antibodies p 222–246

Lomas C, Bruce M, Watt A, Gabra G S, Muller S, Tippett P 1986 Tar+ individuals with anti-D, a new category D^{vii}. Transfusion (Abstract) 26: 560

Melamed M D, Gordon J, Ley S J, Edgar D, Hughes-Jones N C 1985 Senescence of a human lymphoblastoid clone producing anti-Rhesus (D). European Journal of Immunology 15: 742–746

Mollison P L 1983 Blood Transfusion in Clinical Medicine 7th edition. Blackwell, Oxford

Moore S, Woodrow C F, McClelland B L 1982 Isolation of membrane components associated with human red cell antigens Rh(D), (c), (E) and Fy^a. Nature 295: 529–531

Natvig J B, Kunkel H G, Rosenfield R E, Dalton J F, Kochiva S 1976 Idiotypic specificities of anti-Rh antibodies. Journal of Immunology 116: 1536–1538

Nevanlinna H R, Vaino T 1956 The influence of mother-child ABO incompatibility on Rh immunisation. Vox Sanguinis 1: 26–36

Nicolson G L, Masouredis S P, Singer S J 1971 Quantitative two-dimensional ultrastructural distribution of Rh$_o$(D) antigenic sites on human erythrocyte membranes. Proceedings of the National Academy of Science, USA 68: 1416–1420

Paire J, Monestier M, Rigal D, Martel F, Desranges C 1986 Establishment of human cell lines producing anti-D monoclonal antibodies: identification of Rhesus D antigen. Immunology Letters 13: 137–141

Pattengale P K, Smith R W, Gerber P 1973 Selective transformation of B lymphocytes by EB virus. Lancet II: 93–94

Prevention of Rh-haemolytic disease: final results of the 'high-risk' clinical trial 1971 A combined study from centres in England and Baltimore. British Medical Journal 2: 607–609

Prevention of Rh-haemolytic disease: results of a clinical trial 1966 A combined study from centres in England and Baltimore. British Medical Journal 2: 907–914

Race R R, Sanger R, Lawler S D 1948 The Rh D antigen D^u. Annals of Eugenics 14: 171–184

Ridgwell K, Roberts S J, Tanner M J A, Anstee D J 1983 Absence of two membrane components containing extracellular thiol groups in Rh$_{null}$ human erythrocytes. Biochemical Journal 213: 267–269

Ridgwell K, Tanner M J A, Anstee D J 1984 The Rhesus (D) polypeptide is linked to the human erythrocyte cytoskeleton. Federation of European Biochemical Societies letters 174: 7–10

Rochna E, Hughes-Jones N C 1965 The use of purified ^{125}I-labelled anti-globulin in the determination of the number of D antigen sites on red cells of different phenotypes. Vox Sanguinis 10: 675–686

Roder J C, Cole S P C, Atlaw T, Campling B C, McGarry R C, Kozbor D 1985 Human hybridomas and monoclonal antibodies. Plenum Press, New York p 55–67

Rosen A, Gergely P, Jondal M, Klein G, Britton S 1977 Polyclonal Ig production after Epstein-Barr virus infection of human lymphocytes in vitro. Nature 267: 52–54

Schroff R, Foon K, Beatty S, Oldham R, Morgan A 1985 Human anti-murine immunoglobulin responses in patients receiving monoclonal antibody therapy. Cancer Research 45: 879–885

Sinor L T, Brown P J, Evans J P, Plapp P V 1984 The Rh antigen specificity of erythrocyte proteolipid. Transfusion 24: 179–180

Steinitz M, Klein G, Koskimies S, Makela O 1977 EB virus induced B lymphocyte cell live producing specific antibody. Nature 269: 420–422

Steinitz M, Koskimies S, Klein G, Makela O 1979 Establishment of specific antibody producing human lines by antigen preselection and Epstein-Barr (EBV) transformation Clinical and laboratory Immunology 2: 1–7

Steinitz M, Tamir S 1982 Human monoclonal autoimmune antibody produced in vitro: rheumatoid factor generated by Epstein-Barr virus-transformed cell line. European Journal of Immunology 12: 126–133

Stratton F, Renton P H 1948 Rh genes allelomorphic to D. Nature 162:293

Stratton F 1946 A new Rh allelomorph. Nature 158:25

Teng N N H, Lam K S, Riera F C, Kaplan H S 1983 Construction and testing of mouse-human hetero-myelomas for human monoclonal antibody production. Proceedings of the National Academy of Science USA 80: 7308–7312

Teng N N H, Reyes G R, Bieber M D, Fry K E, Lam K S, Herbert J M 1986 Human hybridomas and monoclonal antibodies. Plenum Press, London, p 71–87

Thompson K M, Melamed M D, Eagle K et al 1986 Production of human monoclonal IgG and IgM antibodies with anti-D (rhesus) specificity using heterohybridomas. Immunology 58: 157–160

Tippett P, Sanger R 1977 Further observations on the subdivisions of the Rh antigen Das Arztliche Laboratorium 23: 476–480

Tippett P, Sanger R 1962 Observations on the subdivisions of the Rh antigen D. Vox Sanguinis 7: 9–13

Tovey L A D 1986 Haemolytic disease of the newborn – the changing scene. British Journal of Obstetrics and Gynaecology 93: 960–966

Urbaniak S J 1985 Rh (D) haemolytic disease of the newborn: the changing scene. British Medical Journal 291: 4–6

Voak D, Lennox E, Sacks S, Milstein C, Darnborough J 1982 Monoclonal anti-A and anti-B development as cost-effective reagents. Medical Laboratory Science 39: 109–122

Wiener A S, Unger L J 1962 Further observations on the Rh blood factors Rh^A, Rh^B, Rh^C and Rh^D. Transfusion 2: 230–233

Wiener A S, Peters H R 1940 Hemolytic reactions following transfusions of blood of the homologous group, with three cases in which the same agglutination was responsible. Annals of Internal Medicine 13: 2306–2322

Winger L, Winger C, Shastry P, Russell A, Longenecker M 1983 Efficient generation in vitro of monoclonal Epstein-Barr virus-transformants producing specific antibody to a variety of antigens, without prior deliberate immunisation. Proceedings of the National Academy of Science USA 80: 4484–4488

Woodrow J C, Clarke C A, Donohoe W T A et al 1975 Mechanism of Rh prophylaxis: an experimental study of specificity of immunosuppression. British Medical Journal 2: 57–59

Young W W, Johnson H S, Tamura Y et al 1983 Characterisation of monoclonal antibodies specific for the lewis^a human blood group determinant. Journal of Biological Chemistry 258: 4890–4894

Yvart J, Gerbal A, Cartron J, Salmon C 1974 Etude comparee de divrses methodes de mise en evidence de, l'antigene D^u. Revue, Française Transfusion 17: 201–209

Transfusion support of haemoglobinopathies

INTRODUCTION

Remarkable strides have been made during the past quarter of a century in understanding the molecular biology, genetics, and pathophysiology of abnormal haemoglobins and disordered haemoglobin production. Ironically, the key to medical management of patients with clinically severe haemoglobinopathies remains an 'old' therapy, blood transfusion. However, transfusion practice has hardly remained stagnant during this period. Improved products, methods, and transfusion strategies have evolved in step with new information about the role and effects of transfusion. Unfortunately, progress has not been without its dark side. The benefits of transfusion have been accompanied by life-threatening complications. This chapter will focus on current concepts and problems in the use of blood to support patients with the common, clinically significant haemoglobinopathies.

THE THALASSAEMIA SYNDROMES

The thalassaemias are a heterogeneous group of inherited red cell disorders characterized at the molecular level by decreased or absent synthesis of polypeptide globin chains of the haemoglobin molecule. The individual disorders are classified according to the specific globin chain(s) affected. In patients who are symptomatic, anaemia results from shortened red cell survival, ineffective erythropoiesis, or a combination of these defects. Different complex molecular mechanisms account for the variability in clinical severity among these disorders. Accordingly, the term 'thalassaemia major' is generally used to describe a clinical syndrome and does not necessarily refer to a particular molecular defect or to the zygosity of the defect.

Thalassaemia major is a life-threatening disease which usually becomes apparent in the first year of life. Affected patients are found to be anaemic and lethargic and fail to thrive. These patients subsequently suffer growth retardation and develop hepatosplenomegaly and chronic bone marrow hypertrophy with characteristic skeletal changes on x-ray and pathologic fractures. When untreated, many patients with thalassaemia major die in early childhood from the effects of severe anaemia.

Transfusion

Transfusion therapy in thalassaemia was first used as a life-saving measure; however, indications were soon extended to afford patients symptomatic relief as well. In 1964, a retrospective study of 60 thalassaemic children further demonstrated that those with a higher haemoglobin, and a history of more transfusion, seemed to be in better health and physical condition (Wolman 1964). These observations led to the currently accepted practice of instituting chronic prophylactic transfusion for patients whose haemoglobin level remains below 7 g/dl or who show evidence of growth retardation or skeletal alteration at a haemoglobin above this level. Subsequently, the trend has been to maintain such patients at increasingly higher mean haemoglobin levels.

The 'hypertransfusion regimen' introduced in 1969 was designed to depress endogenous erythropoiesis and prevent bone marrow hypertrophy (Piomelli et al 1969). According to this regimen, haemoglobin concentration is maintained at a minimum level of 10 g/dl and a mean level of 12 g/dl. Although hypertransfusion failed to suppress endogenous erythropoiesis entirely and did not prevent hypersplenism, it did improve growth and development during the first decade of life and importantly, reduced endogenous iron absorption and skeletal deformity in thalassaemic children (Necheles et al 1974, de Alarcon et al 1979).

A transfusion regimen known as 'supertransfusion', proposed in 1980, was reported to shrink the pathologically expanded bone marrow and thereby reduce blood volume and eventually transfusion requirement in thalassaemia major (Propper et al 1980). Supertransfusion maintains the minimum haemoglobin level at 12 g/dl and the mean between 14 and 15 g/dl. The benefits of this regimen have not been adequately tested, and certainly not proved. Preliminary reports suggest that to the contrary, increasing the minimum haemoglobin level may not reduce transfusion requirement as predicted, but may in fact increase the use of blood and the resultant iron deposition (Piomelli et al 1980, Modell et al 1984). These apparently contradictory findings reported from different centres may be partially reconciled by the observation that patients with different thalassaemia syndromes have varying levels of endogenous erythropoiesis. Red cell production may influence both the amount of transfusion needed to maintain a given haemoglobin level and the iron excretion response to chelation therapy (Pippard et al 1982). Until these issues are clarified, physicians who elect to use a supertransfusion regimen should monitor blood use and iron accumulation closely.

Splenectomy still plays an important role in the transfusion management of thalassaemia. Although chronic transfusion delays the progression of hepatosplenomegaly, no regimen yet has prevented the development of hypersplenism. Splenic destruction of transfused red cells may increase the transfusion requirement significantly. Neither spleen size nor clinical studies of spleen function accurately predicts the degree of hypersplenism. The best indication that splenectomy will benefit the patient is a progressively increasing transfusion requirement, especially one that approaches the range of 230 ml/kg packed red cells per year. At this point, usually before age 10 in patients with thalassaemia major, splenectomy may reduce transfusion requirement by up to 75% (Cohen et al 1985, Piomelli et al 1985).

Red cell preparations

Red cell concentrates ('packed' red cells) are the standard component used in transfusion programmes for thalassaemic patients. Because refrigerated red cell storage results in a progressive decline in red cell diphosphoglycerate (DPG) and increased oxygen affinity, some centres prefer to use red cells which are either less than six days old or stored in the frozen state. However, red cells drawn from transfusion-dependent thalassaemic patients contain unexpectedly low levels of DPG (Correra et al 1984). Ordinarily, stored red cells totally depleted of DPG would be expected to regenerate DPG within hours of transfusion. Since neither the cause of this finding in thalassaemic patients nor its physiologic significance is known, it seems premature to stipulate a special red cell product solely for its DPG level.

Red cell concentrates may be modified to prevent the immune-mediated reactions commonly encountered in chronically transfused patients. Recurrent febrile reactions caused by antigenic determinants on leukocytes contained in the red cell preparation are related to the number of contaminant leukocytes (Perkins et al 1966). While several methods can remove sufficient leukocytes to prevent these reactions, microaggregate filtration is the simplest and effective technique and has the further virtue of minimizing red cell loss and cost (Meryman et al 1986). Less frequently and less predictably, allergic reactions to plasma components complicate chronic transfusion. Although red cells can be saline-washed relatively free of plasma and leukocytes, there is an attendant loss of red cells in the process. Washed red cells must be transfused within 24 hours of preparation. For the severely sensitized patient, it may be necessary to resort to frozen-deglycerolyzed red cells, a preparation virtually free of other contaminating blood components, but time-consuming to prepare, expensive, and importantly a product which may increase the transfusion requirement significantly (Piomelli et al 1974). Neither washed nor frozen cells should be used routinely, but should be reserved for patients with documented transfusion reactions.

Young red cells

In many areas of the world, the high infant mortality previously associated with untransfused thalassaemia major has been replaced by a rising adolescent mortality caused by the complications of transfusion iron overload. Every 1 ml of red cells deposits 1.08 mg iron in tissues as the red cells are catabolized. Serious cardiac dysfunction in thalassaemic patients occurs at a body iron burden of about 20 g, the equivalent of 100 units of blood (Buja et al 1971). Because the iron content of a red cell is independent of the cell's age, an 'old' transfused cell, which might survive but a few hours in the recipient, will deposit as much iron as a 'young' cell which might survive several months. In theory, units of young red cells should decrease transfusion frequency and ultimately delay the accumulation of iron in regularly transfused patients.

The observation that red cell density increases with age and that gradient techniques can isolate young red cells on the basis of their buoyant density suggested a practical method for collecting units of young cells for transfusion (Piomelli et al 1978). Initial attempts to collect such units from single donors by means of continuous flow cell separators demonstrated the feasibility of this approach (Propper et al 1980, Corash et al 1981). While units collected in this fashion show prolonged red cell survival in vivo, they are extremely difficult to collect, smaller than standard units, and prohibitively expensive. Technical innovations have made the isolation of young red cells easier and less costly. A cell washer technique (Bracey et al 1983, Graziano et al 1982) and a filtration-centrifugation method using standard, commercially available equipment (Hogan et al 1986) permit separation of the 'young third' from whole blood donations. Each procedure requires the use of two to three modified units to equal the haemoglobin content of a standard unit, thus increasing patient exposure to multiple donors.

Clinical information confirming long-term transfusion benefit from young red cell products is both limited and disappointing. Cell-washer preparations have been used to support patients in three centres. The most successful programme reports that in six chronically transfused, splenectomized patients followed for one year, transfusion requirement declined an average of 15.8%, far less than had been predicted (Cohen et al 1984). The other centres, with an aggregate of 55 patients, report insufficient reduction in transfusion requirement to justify either the exposure of patients to additional donor risk or the added expense (Piomelli et al 1985, Marcus et al 1985). Clinical studies have not yet been performed with the filtration-centrifugation product.

An intriguing theoretical approach to the chronic transfusion-iron overload problem involves placing the patient on a cell separator to remove old cells while transfusing with young cells, a true red cell exchange. Such a technique has been employed for one patient whose reported transfusion requirement fell remarkably from 160 mg/kg haemoglobin per year to

74 mg/kg haemoglobin per year while on this programme (Wolfe et al 1985). Few details of this patient's transfusion experience have been published. Before routine use of young red cells can be recommended, confirmation of this report or similar evidence of clinical success needs to be forthcoming. For the present, transfusion of young red cells in managing thalassaemia remains an investigational practice.

SICKLE CELL DISEASE

Sickle cell disease encompasses a group of inherited disorders in which a mutation in the globin gene results in production of the abnormal haemoglobin, S. Clinical sickling disorders are seen with a variety of genotypes including SS, SC, S-β thalassaemia, but not with 'sickle trait' (AS) and many other mixed heterozygous states. Even among patients homozygous for the sickle gene, there is a wide spectrum of clinical illness. The most severely affected patients develop marked anaemia and widespread organ dysfunction as a result of vaso-occlusion. Complications include transient aplasia, stroke, pulmonary infarction, priapism, recurrent abortion, aseptic necrosis of a variety of bones, and the much publicized painful crises.

The pathogenesis of sickle cell disease is poorly understood. At the molecular level, deoxyhemoglobin S undergoes polymerization within the red cell making the cell rigid and poorly deformable. Polymer formation is most likely to occur in organs where sluggish capillary blood flow and conditions of temperature and pH predispose to deoxygenation, such as in the kidney and in the spleen. Intracellular haemoglobin gel formation may prevent ready transit of the red cell through capillary beds even before the cell assumes the characteristic sickle shape and this may result in tissue ischaemia and necrosis (Noguchi et al 1981). It is not clear that local increases in whole blood viscosity related to sickling or increased adhesion of sickle cells to endothelial cells play an important role in large and small vessel vaso-occlusion. The chronic haemolysis seen in the sickle cell syndromes is probably even less important as a cause of disease.

Transfusion therapy

Transfusion therapy can correct the anaemia associated with sickle cell disease when it is deemed desirable to do so. In addition, by diluting the patient's abnormal red cells with transfused cells, whole blood viscosity and rheology are favorably altered. As few as 30% transfused cells markedly decrease viscosity when measured with an Ostwald viscometer and resistance to membrane filterability approaches normal at mixtures of 50% and above (Anderson et al 1963, Lessin et al 1978). The critical issue for clinicians remains whether transfusion alters the underlying course of sickle cell disease, and if not, whether it favourably modifies complications or symptoms. For each patient, the goals or transfusion should be outlined and an appropriate transfusion programme designed. Chronic transfusion should never be undertaken without specific indications.

There is experimental evidence to support the use of transfusion in treating sickle cell disease. First, transfusion of four infants with sickle cell anaemia and a renal concentrating defect restored renal concentrating ability to normal (Keitel et al 1956). However, the concentrating defect in a 10 year old child reversed only slowly and incompletely, and two adults recovered no renal concentrating ability. Correlation of the reversibility with age has been confirmed, suggesting that in the kidney at least, the initial defect is a functional one, but that eventually an irreversible structural change takes place (Statius van Eps et al 1967). Second, in five children with functional asplenia, transfusion restored splenic reticuloendothelial function, although transiently (Pearson et al 1970). All five patients were found to have splenomegaly on physical examination. Third, both transfusion and exchange transfusion have improved exercise tolerance in a small series of patients, even when post exchange haemoglobin elevation was minimal (Miller et al 1980, Charache et al 1983). Finally, large periodic, local oscillations in cutaneous blood flow, characteristic of sickle cell disease, can be reversed by exchange transfusion (Rodgers et al 1984). Caution must be exercised, however, in using such findings to draw conclusions about the role of transfusion in preventing sickle pain crises, or in otherwise modifying the natural history of sickle cell disease.

When transfusion is indicated, the guidelines for red cell preparation and transfusion are similar to those followed for patients with thalassaemia and for other chronically transfused patients. In addition, it is prudent to avoid using blood from donors with sickle trait, since these donor cells may sickle should the patient become hypoxic, and their presence obscures accurate calculation of the percentage of transfused cells. Determinations of haemoglobin concentration and quantitative haemoglobin electrophoresis should be performed on samples prior to and post-transfusion to follow the effectiveness of the procedure. While no clinical data support a single ideal level of transfusion, most centres try to maintain the haemoglobin A level above 50% and the haemoglobin concentration in the 10–12 g/dl range for their transfused patients. High levels of haemoglobin A are easily achieved in a chronic transfusion programme because of the combination of marrow suppression and the selective survival advantage of the transfused cells.

Exchange transfusion

Partial exchange transfusion was introduced more than 20 years ago. The advantages of the exchange technique are: 1. a high level of transfused cells can be reached relatively quickly; 2. dangerous elevations in blood volume and haemoglobin concentration can be avoided; 3. for patients who require chronic transfusion, iron accumulation is delayed. The first manual exchanges consisted of a 500 ml phlebotomy followed by a two unit transfusion, and achieved about a 30% red cell exchange (Anderson et al 1963). Larger volume manual exchange procedures required placement of indwelling venous catheters and employed systemic anticoagulation. Still another approach involved an alternate phlebotomy-transfusion regimen carried out over several days. All of these techniques effectively exchange red cells, but are tedious, labour intensive and may result in dangerous oscillations in the patient's blood volume.

The first automated red cell exchange was performed on a continuous-flow centrifugal cell separator, provided a 90% exchange in $3\frac{1}{2}$ h, and did not result in any obvious adverse effects (Kernoff et al 1977). Since that time, several thousand exchange procedures have been performed safely and easily on a variety of commercial instruments. A six unit exchange will bring the haemoglobin A level of the average untransfused adult to 50% or above and can be completed in less than 90 minutes (Klein et al 1980). Automated exchange is easily performed in an outpatient setting and requires minimal personnel time, partially offsetting its additional cost compared to manual exchange.

The volume and frequency of red cell exchange remain controversial. While in vitro studies suggest that as little as 30–50% exchange should be effective, some patients remain symptomatic when maintained at levels of 80% normal haemoglobin and above. Such failures may be due in part to pre-existing irreversible ischaemic organ damage. For any given procedure, the amount of blood exchanged to reach a desired level depends on the patient's size, haemoglobin concentration, and percent haemoglobin S prior to exchange. Elegant formulae have been derived to predict the haemoglobin S concentration at any time during the procedure (Alcuri 1985). This degree of precision hardly seems necessary. The average adult will require about 5 units every six weeks to keep the haemoglobin concentration above 10 g/dl and the haemoglobin A above the 50% level. The exchange schedule can be modified based on actual measurements. The patient's final haematocrit can be easily altered during the procedure by using packed red cells instead of whole blood and by manipulating the force of the centrifugal path by altering bowl speed.

The age and storage conditions of the replacement red cells do not appear to be important. An early report raised concerns about rapid replacement of cells with elevated DPG levels in sickle-cell patients with banked blood depleted of DPG (White et al 1976). For this reason frozen, deglycerolized cells were often preferred because of their superior oxygen delivery characteristics. However, the initial fears appear to be unfounded. The change in oxygen affinity induced acutely by exchange transfusion is probably of little physiologic significance compared with the improved oxygen delivery properties of blood when sickle cells are replaced with normal cells (Miller et al 1980). There is no evidence that refrigerated, stored red cells are any less effective clinically. Since refrigerated cells do contain aggregates of platelet and leukocyte debris, an in-line fine filter ($20–40\mu$) placed in the return line is a useful precaution. When several units of refrigerated cells are to be exchanged rapidly, an in-line blood warmer is recommended as well.

One attractive possibility of automated red cell exchange is the selective removal of sickle cells. Irreversibly sickled cells are much denser than normal red cells and should be differentially sedimented in a centrifugal field. Preliminary studies have been encouraging (Lenes et al 1983). However, irreversibly sickled cells do not often circulate in large numbers and their presence does not correlate well with clinical disease. Most of the cells containing haemoglobin S are in fact younger and lighter than the transfused cells. It is likely that technical modifications of the available cell separator rotors will be necessary before this approach becomes practical.

Clinical indications for transfusion

Aplastic crises are among the few non-controversial indications for transfusing patients with sickle cell disease. Transient bone marrow suppression may follow relatively mild infections, especially those caused by the parvovirus, and life-threatening anaemia may result (Young et al 1984). Cautious transfusion should be dictated by the clinical situation. Although severe, the anaemia is temporary and there is no need to continue transfusion once marrow recovery is reflected by reticulocytosis. Transfusion does not appear to delay or impair marrow recovery.

Sudden, severe anaemia in childhood may be accompanied by massive enlargement of the spleen. The 'splenic sequestration crisis' accounts for a substantial number of early deaths in patients with sickle cell disease (Topley et al 1981). In striking contrast to the aplastic crisis, the sequestration crisis is usually accompanied by hypotension. Therefore, immediate treatment consists of transfusion of whole blood or of red cells and volume expanders. Although the sequestration crisis responds dramatically to appropriate therapy, patients tend to have recurrent episodes, so that continued prophylactic transfusion is often recommended (Cohen 1985).

Since blood oxygenation is the most critical factor in the management of patients with sickling haemoglobinopathies, failure to treat pulmonary problems early and aggressively may have disastrous consequences. Many patients who present with pulmonary symptoms and little objective evidence of pulmonary disease progress to develop fever, tachypnea, pulmonary infiltrates and severe respiratory distress, a complex which has come to be known as the 'acute chest syndrome.' Often the cause of the pulmonary infiltrates is never determined. From a number of case reports and large retrospective series, there is convincing evidence that intravascular sickling accounts for much of the clinical problem (Davies et al 1984b). Response to exchange transfusion is frequently dramatic, often with resolution of symptoms within 24 hours. Regardless of the cause of acute chest syndrome, sickle cell patients with rapidly worsening respiratory distress should undergo exchange transfusion as part of their overall management.

Priapism is an unusual but well-recognized acute complication of sickle cell disease. Although most episodes resolve within 24 hours, as many as a third of patients with recurrent priapism eventually become impotent (Emond et al 1980). The results of surgical intervention are hardly encouraging. Although the reported effectiveness of transfusion and exchange transfusion in relieving priapism is strictly anecdotal, both seem reasonable approaches for patients with persistent, painful erection (Kinney et al 1975). Our own experience with five patients suggests that transfusion is most effective when performed early in an episode and for patients who have had few previous episodes. Exchange transfusion to levels of 90% occasionally appears to help when less extensive exchanges fail.

Painful crises are characterized by abdominal and bone pain, fever and myalgias. Most patients can define a pattern specific to their pain crises, but there is no diagnostic test to indicate the presence or severity of such crises. The role of transfusion in these vaso-occlusive pain crises is controversial. Small series report the effectiveness of exchange transfusion in shortening vaso-occlusive episodes (Brody et al 1970, Green et al 1975), however, there is no convincing evidence that raising the haematocrit or lowering the percentage of haemoglobin S predictably shortens or decreases the severity of painful crises. Prophylactic chronic transfusion may prevent or lessen the frequency of painful crises in patients who have recurrent episodes (Anderson et al 1963, Cohen 1985). Such a programme is worth consideration for patients whose quality of life is severely impaired by recurrent pain. However, clinical manifestations of sickle cell disease vary greatly with time and there is little objective information to support routine chronic exchange therapy to prevent painful crises. It is unlikely that these issues will be settled without carefully controlled studies.

Up to 10% of children with sickle cell disease will suffer stroke and, if untreated, up to two-thirds will have additional central nervous system episodes (Powars et al 1978). In a series of 30 patients with sickle cell disease and acute neurologic episodes, 23 had multiple abnormalities of major cerebral arteries shown by arteriography (Russell et al 1984). Chronic transfusion therapy substantially reduced the progression of vascular changes when compared with studies of four untransfused patients. Stroke was reduced to 10% compared to the 90% recurrence rate experienced in this patient population prior to transfusion therapy. The most practical regimen is probably an exchange transfusion programme where the level of haemoglobin S is kept below 50%. Although such a programme seems clearly indicated for patients who have sustained a stroke, the period of such therapy and the risk at the time of cessation are not well defined.

No controlled studies compare morbidity and mortality of transfused patients with sickle cell disease who require surgery with that of untransfused control patients. The case for prophylactic preoperative transfusion or exchange transfusion rests on case reports and on the uncontrolled observations at different centres. Not surprisingly, the published experience varies widely. At one institution more than 200 consecutive procedures requiring general anaesthesia were performed on patients with sickling disorders and no significant complications were seen (Homi et al 1980). In contrast, a review of 144 patients with sickling disorders revealed 11 deaths after general anaesthesia; several of these may well have been prevented by prophylactic transfusion (Searle 1973). Because the patients, their clinical status, an institution's surgical facilities and experience, as well as many other factors are not equivalent, the apparent contradictions in these and other reports are understandable.

The rationale for preoperative transfusion is that general anaesthesia poses an increased risk for patients with sickling haemoglobinopathies. A short period of accidental hypoxia has little consequence for most patients, but may result in generalized sickling for these subjects. In addition, other hazzards of surgery and the postoperative period, such as acidosis, hypothermia, hypotension, dehydration, and postoperative pneumonitis, would appear to place the sickle cell patient at increased risk. While it is not clear that transfusion reduces this risk, several large series report minimal postoperative problems related to sickling when patients are transfused or exchanged pre-operatively (Morrison et al 1978, Fullerton et al 1982). Although patients with uncomplicated surgical procedures probably benefit little from preoperative transfusion, reducing the level of haemoglobin S below 50% may well provide a margin of safety, especially when the procedure or recovery run less smoothly than anticipated.

Sickle cell disease greatly complicates pregnancy. Not only are maternal problems of pregnancy such as pre-eclampsia, pulmonary embolism, urinary tract infection, and congestive heart failure more likely to occur in these patients, but spontaeous abortion and intrauterine growth retardation become major fetal risks (Sergeant 1983). As in the case of general anesthesia, several large uncontrolled studies support the use of blood transfusion to decrease maternal morbidity and improve fetal salvage, but differences in study design, patient population, and prenatal care make these reports difficult to compare and evaluate (Morrison et al 1980, Cunningham et al 1983). With careful prenatal care, some centres report few fetal and maternal problems when transfusions are restricted to those patients whose clinical condition worsens significantly during pregnancy (Charache et al 1985). However, most clinicians have concluded that regular transfusion begun early in pregnancy results in minimal maternal morbidity and fetal loss, with few complications from the transfusion programme.

The goal of most centres that initiate a prophylactic transfusion programme is to keep the percentage of transfused cells above 50%. This goal is easily achieved by simple transfusion if the patient is begun early in pregnancy and evaluated regularly. For those patients who present late in pregnancy, partial exchange transfusion may be required, and if complications of sickle cell disease persist, many centres will use this technique to increase the percentage of transfused cells to 80% or more.

Summary

Transfusion is a useful therapeutic procedure in managing sickle cell disease. At present, its major role lies in treating the acute complications of the disease such as the aplastic crisis and the acute chest syndrome. In other acute conditions, such as priapism, retinal artery occlusion, and severe painful crisis, the effectiveness of transfusion or partial exchange is less clear, but in the absence of effective alternative treatment, transfusion is a reasonable approach.

There is increasing evidence that transfusion plays an important prophylactic role in selected patients. For those patients who have suffered stroke, transfusion decreases the risk of a subsequent event, although the degree and length of prophylactic transfusion remain unclear. Prenatal and presurgical transfusion are clearly useful for certain high-risk patients with sickle cell disease, and may benefit the majority of patients in these situations. There is little evidence to support a role for routine transfusion in preventing infections, painful crises, cardiac disease, degenerative bone disease, chronic ankle ulcers or in altering the underlying course of the patient with a sickling haemoglobinopathy. Since the clinical manifestations of sickle cell disease tend to vary with time, it is unlikely that any of these questions will be answered without carefully controlled studies.

COMPLICATIONS OF TRANSFUSION

Patients with haemoglobin disorders are subject to all the hazards associated with blood transfusion. However, certain complications take on increased importance, either because they are more likely to cause problems for chronically transfused subjects, or because their effects are peculiar to this patient group.

Regular transfusion causes progressive accumulation of iron, leading to cellular damage and ultimately to death. In patients with thalassaemia major, life-span is now determined by the rate of myocardial iron deposition with death occurring as a result of intractable heart failure or arrhythmia, usually between the ages of 15 and 25 years (Ley et al 1982). Iron accumulates in virtually all tissues of the body. Although transfusional iron overload appears to be less of a problem in patients with sickle cell disease, it can occur when these patients are placed on chronic transfusion programmes (Davies et al 1984a).

The only effective means of removing iron in transfusion dependent patients is by use of the iron chelating agent, desferoxamine. Aggressive chelation therapy of patients with thalassaemia major, when begun in childhood, appears to prevent cardiac iron accumulation and reduce mortality

(Modell et al 1982). Sickle cell patients on a chronic partial exchange transfusion programme remain in positive iron balance, but accumulation is so slow that chelation is rarely required. Nevertheless, all chronically transfused patients should be closely monitored for evidence of iron accumulation and treated before clinical evidence of toxicity occurs.

The large number of donor exposures places patients with transfusion supported haemoglobinopathies at substantial risk of contracting hepatitis and other blood-borne infections. Although death from acute hepatitis or cirrhosis is uncommon, as many as 25% of transfused patients with thalassaemia show evidence of exposure to hepatitis B viral markers and 80% to other markers of hepatitis (Moroni et al 1984). Morbidity and mortality from exposure to hepatotropic viruses is likely to increase as deaths in childhood and adolescence from other causes decline. Although few reports of transfusion-related acquired immune deficiency syndrome (AIDS) have yet been published in this patient group, more than 10% of patients in one large study showed evidence of exposure to HIV, the implicated viral agent (De Martino et al 1985). Finally, an increasing number of reports document such nonspecific evidence of immunologic abnormality as altered lymphocyte subtypes, cutaneous energy, reduced mitogen response and nonfunctional natural killer cells in chronically transfused patients. Whether these changes are related to transfusion-transmitted viruses and whether they will have clinical significance remains to be seen.

Alloimmunization can be a serious problem in chronically transfused patients. Although estimates vary, up to a third of these patients may develop alloantibodies and at least one report failed to find a significant difference in frequency between transfused sickle cell patients and those with thalassaemia (Coles et al 1981). Occasional patients with thalassaemia succumb to severe anaemia when compatible blood can no longer be found. There is currently no effective solution for this problem in thalassaemia. Recently, sickle red cells have successfully been frozen, enabling a sickle cell patient with multiple alloantibodies and no compatible donors to donate 11 autologous units in preparation for elective surgery (Chaplin et al 1986).

Another potentially important consequence of red cell alloimmunization is delayed immune haemolysis. Although in most patients this complication is usually mild and often scarcely detected if not for mild temperature elevation and poor response to transfusion, in sickle cell patients, especially when exchange transfused, such reactions may masquerade as severe, even life threatening vaso-occlusive crises (Diamond et al 1980). Whether the severity of the reaction is related to the large volume of incompatible blood present, to the presence of the remaining sickle cells, or to other factors, is not clear. However, since the common laboratory indicators of haemolysis may be masked by the patient's chronic haemolytic state, a high index of suspicion must be entertained when a recently transfused sickle cell patient returns in crisis. Further transfusion should be withheld until immune haemolysis has been ruled out.

The advantages and disadvantage of extended red cell phenotyping have been debated (Diamond et al 1980, Blumberg et al 1984). At the very least, this practice is helpful in identifying immune mediated haemolysis should a reaction occur. In view of the potentially dire consequences of delayed haemolysis in sickle cell patients, it seems prudent and relatively inexpensive to match red cells for the common clinically important antigens (Rh, Kell, Kidd, Duffy) for those patients who have identified themselves as immunologic 'responders' by producing red cell alloantibodies. Routine use of extended 'phenotype identical' blood is unwarranted.

A rare but potentially fatal encephalopathy has been reported as a result of transfusion in both sickle cell patients and thalassaemics (Royal et al 1978, Wasi et al 1978). The syndrome is characterized by headaches, hypertension, seizures and cerebral hemorrhage. It has been postulated that vasoactive substances in the transfusions cause these events, but there is little evidence to support this idea. Although it is unlikely that the syndrome is related to whole blood hyperviscosity, exchange transfusion has been recommended for sickle cell patients who develop evidence of encephalopathy. It is probably more important to recognize the significance of hypertension and headaches when these patients are transfused and treat early and aggressively.

CONCLUSION

Although haemoglobin disorders are prototype molecular diseases in an era of molecular biology, tranfusion remains the major form of therapy in managing the symptomatic haemoglobinopathies. There is little question that transfusion has extended the life of patients with thalassaemia major and improved the quality of life both for these patients and for many patients with sickling haemoglobinopathies. Less frequently, patients with milder forms of thalassaemia and with rare unstable haemoglobins benefit from transfusion therapy as well. Improved red cell products, transfusion strategies, laboratory methods, and instrumentation, have made transfusion support increasingly safe, easy, and inexpensive. Despite the hazards of chronic transfusion, blood is likely to remain the most effective therapy for haemoglobin disorders until the molecular defect can be corrected by some more basic approach.

REFERENCES

Alcuri S J 1985 A mathematical model for exchange red blood cell apheresis using a continuous-flow automated blood cell separator. Plasma Therapy and Transfusion Technology 6: 761–769

Anderson R, Cassell M, Mullinax G L et al 1963 Effect of normal cells on viscosity of sickle-cell blood: In vitro studies and report of six years experience with a prophylactic programme of 'partial exchange transfusion.' Archives of Internal Medicine 111: 286–294

Blumberg N, Ross K, Avila E 1984 Should chronic transfusion be matched for antigens other than ABO and Rh(o)D? Vox Sanguinis 47: 205–208

Bracey A W , Klein H G, Chambers S et al 1983 Ex vivo selective isolation of young red blood cells using the IBM 2991 cell washer. Blood 61: 1068–1071

Brody J I, Goldsmith M H, Park S K et al 1970 Symptomatic crises of sickle cell anemia treated by limited exchange transfusion. Annals of Internal Medicine 72: 327–330

Buja L M, Roberts W C 1971 Iron in the heart: Etiology and clinical significance. American Journal of Medicine 51: 209–221

Chaplin H Jr, Mischeaux J R, Inkster M D et al 1986 Frozen autologous storage of 11 units of sickle cell red cells for autologous transfusion of a sickle cell patient. Transfusion 26: 341–345

Charache E, Niebyl J R 1985 Pregnancy in sickle cell disease. Clinics in Haematology 14: 729–746

Charache S, Bleeker E R, Bross D S 1983 Effects of blood transfusion on exercise capacity in patients with sickle-cell anemia. American Journal of Medicine 74: 757–764

Cohen A R, Schmidt J M, Martin M B et al 1984 Clinical trial of young red cell transfusion. Journal of Pediatrics 104: 865–868

Cohen A R 1985 Transfusion therapy for children and adolescents with hemoglobin disorders. Hemotherapy in Childhood and Adolescence. Arlington: American Association of Blood Banks

Coles S M, Klein H G, Holland P V 1981 Alloimmunization in two multitransfused patient populations. Transfusion 21: 462–466

Corash L, Klein H, Deisseroth A et al 1981 Selective isolation of young erythrocytes for transfusion support of thalassemia major patients. Blood 57: 599–606

Correra A, Graziano J H, Seaman C 1984 Inappropriately low red cell 2, 3-diphosphoglycerate and p50 in transfused-thalassemia. Blood 63: 803–806

Cunningham F G, Pritchard J A, Mason R 1983 Pregnancy and sickle hemoglobinopathies: results with and without prophylactic transfusion. Obstetrics and Gynecology 62: 419–424

Davies S, Henthorn J S, Winn J A et al 1984a Effect of blood transfusion on iron status in sickle cell anemia. Clinical Laboratory Haematology 6: 7–22

Davies S C, Luce P J, Winn A A et al 1984b Acute chest syndrome in sickle cell disease. Lancet 1: 36–38

de Alarcon P A, Donovan M, Forbes G B et al 1979 Iron absorption in the thalassemia syndromes and its inhibition by tea. New England Journal of Medicine 300: 5–8

De Martino M, Quarta G, Melpignano A et al 1985 Antibodies to HTLV-III and the lymphadenopathy syndrome in multitransfused beta-thalassemia patients. Vox Sanguinis 49: 230–233

Diamond W J, Brown F L Jr, Bitterman P et al 1980 Delayed hemolytic transfusion reaction presenting as sickle cell crisis. Annals of Internal Medicine 93: 231–233

Emond A M, Holman R, Hayes R J et al 1980 Priapism and impotence in sickle cell disease. Archives of Internal Medicine 140: 1434

Fullerton M W, Philippart A I, Sarnaik S et al 1982 Preoperative exchange transfusion in sickle cell anemia. Journal of Pediatric Surgery 16: 297–300

Graziano J H, Piomelli S, Seaman C et al 1982 A simple technique for preparation of young red cells for transfusion from ordinary blood units

Green M, Hall R J C, Huntsman R G et al 1975 Sickle cell crisis treated by exchange transfusion. Treatment of two patients with heterozygous sickle cell syndrome. Journal of the American Medical Association 231: 948–950

Hogan V A, Blanchette V S, Rock G 1986 A simple method for preparing neocyte-enriched leukocyte poor blood for transfusion dependent patients. Transfusion 26: 253–257

Homi J, Sergeant G R 1980 General anaesthesia in sickle cell disease. Pediatrics 65:861

Keitel H G, Thompson D, Itano H A 1956 Hyposthenuria in sickle anemia: a reversible defect. Journal of Clinical Investigation 35:998

Kernoff L M, Botha M C, Jacobs P 1977 Exchange transfusion in sickle cell disease using a continuous-flow blood cell separator. Transfusion 17: 269–271

Kinney T R, Harris M B, Russell M O et al 1975 Priapism in association with sickle hemoglobinopathies in children. Journal of Pediatrics 86: 241–242

Klein H G, Garner R J, Miller D M et al 1980 Automated partial exchange transfusion in sickle cell anemia. Transfusion 20: 578–584

Lenes B, Klein H G, Lakatos E 1983 Selective removal of sickle cells with the IBM 2997 continuous flow blood cell separator. Journal of Clinical Apheresis 1: 64–70

Lessin L S, Kurantsin-Mills J, Klug P P et al 1978 Determination of rheologically optimal mixtures of AA and SS erythrocytes for transfusion. Progress in Clinical and Biological Research 20: 123–137

Ley T J, Griffith P, Nienhuis A W 1982 Transfusional hemosiderosis and chelation therapy. Clinics in Hematology 11:437

Marcus R E, Wonke B , Bantock H M et al 1985 A prospective trial of young red cells in 48 patients with transfusion-dependent thalassemia. British Journal of Haematology 60: 153–159

Meryman H T, Hornblower M 1986 The preparation of red cells depleted of leukocytes. Transfusion 26: 101–106

Miller D M, Winslow R M, Klein H G 1980 Improved exercise performance after exchange transfusion in subjects with sickle cell anemia. Blood 56: 1127–1131

Modell B, Berdoukas V 1984 The Clinical Approach to Thalassemia. London: Grune and Stratton

Modell E, Letsky E A, Flynn D M et al 1982 Survival and deferoxamine in thalassemia major. British Medical Journal 284: 1081–1084

Moroni G A, Piacentini G, Terzoli S et al 1984 Hepatitis B or non-A, non-B virus infection in multitransfused thalassemic patients. Archives of Disease of Childhood 59: 1127–1130

Morrison J C, Whybrew W D, Bucovaz E T 1978 The use of partial exchange transfusion preoperatively in patients with sickle hemoglobinopathies. American Journal of Obstetrics and Gynecology 132: 59–63

Morrison J C, Schneider J M, Whybrew W D et al 1980 Prophylactic transfusions in patients with sickle hemoglobinopathies: benefit versus risk. Obstetrics and Gynecology 56: 274–280

Necheles T S, Chung S, Sabbah R et al 1974 Intensive transfusion therapy in thalassemia major: an 8-year follow-up. Annals of the New York Academy of Sciences 232: 179–185

Noguchi C T, Schechter A N 1981 The intracellular polymerization of sickle hemoglobin and its relevance to sickle cell disease. Blood 58: 1057–1061

Pearson H A, Cornelius E A, Schwartz A D 1970 Transfusion-reversible functional asplenia in young children with sickle-cell anemia. New England Journal of Medicine 283: 334–337

Perkins H A, Payne R, Ferguson J et al 1966 Nonhemolytic febrile transfusion reactions, Quantitative effects of blood components with emphasis on isoantigenic incompatibility of leukocytes. Vox Sanguinis 11: 578–586

Piomelli S, Danoff S J, Becker M H et al 1969 Prevention of bone malformations and cardiomegaly in Cooley's anemia by early hypertransfusion regimen. Annals of the New York Academy of Sciences 165: 427–436

Piomelli S, Karpatkin M H, Arzanian M et al 1974 Hypertransfusion regimen in patients with Cooley's anemia. Annals of the New York Academy of Sciences 232: 186–192

Piomelli S, Seaman C, Reibman J et al 1978 Separation of younger red cells with improved survival in vivo: An approach to chronic transfusion therapy. Proceedings of the National Academy of Science 75: 3474–3478

Piomelli S, Graziano J, Karpatkin M et al 1980 Chelation therapy, transfusion requirement, and iron balance in young thalassemic patients. Annals of the New York Academy of Science 344: 409–417

Piomelli S, Hart D, Graziano J et al 1985 Current strategies in the management of Cooley's anemia. Annals of the New York Academy of Science 445: 256–267

Pippard M J, Callender S T, Finch C A 1982 Ferrioxamine excretion in iron-loaded man. Blood 60: 288–294

Powars D, Wilson B, Imbus C, et al 1978 The natural history of stroke in sickle cell disease. American Journal of Medicine 65: 461–471

Propper R D, Button L N & Nathan D G 1980 New approaches to the transfusion management of thalassemia. Blood 55: 55–60

Rodgers G P, Schechter A N, Noguchi C T et al 1984 Periodic microcirculatory flow in patients with sickle cell disease. New England Journal of Medicine 311: 1534–1538

Royal J E, Seeler R A 1978 Hypertension, convulsions, and cerebral hemorrhage in sickle cell patients after blood transfusions. Lancet 2:1207

Russell M O, Goldberg H I, Hodson A 1984 Effect of transfusion therapy on arteriographic abnormalities and on recurrence of stroke in sickle cell disease. Blood 63: 162–169

Searle J F 1973 Anaesthesia in sickle cell states. Anaesthesia 28: 48–58

Sergeant G R 1983 Sickle haemoglobin and pregnancy. British Medical Journal 287: 628–630

Statius van Eps I W, Schouten H, la Porte-Wijsman L W et al 1967 The influence of red blood cell transfusions on the hyposthenuria and renal hemodynamics of sickle cell anemia. Clinica Chimica Acta 17: 449–461

Topley J M, Rogers D W, Stevens M C G et al 1981 Acute splenic sequestration and hypersplenism in the first five years in homozygous sickle cell disease. Archives of Disease in Childhood 56: 765–769

Wasi P, Pootrakul P, Piankijagum A et al 1978 A syndrome of hypertension, convulsion and cerebral hemorrhage in thalassemic patients after multiple blood transfusion. Lancet 2: 602–604

White J M, White Y S, Buskard N et al 1976 Increasing whole blood oxygen affinity during rapid exchange transfusion: a potential hazzard. Transfusion, 16: 232–236

Wolfe L, Sallan D, Nathan D G 1985 Current therapy and new approaches to the treatment of thalassemia major. Annals of the New York Academy of Sciences 445: 248–255

Wolman I J 1964 Transfusion therapy in Cooley's anemia: growth and health as related to long-range hemoglobin levels. A progress report. Annals of the New York Academy of Sciences 119: 736–747

Young N S, Mortimer P P, Moore J G et al 1984 Characterization of a virus that causes transient aplastic crises. Journal of Clinical Investigation 73: 224–230

Index